# The Young Mother

## BY WM. A. ALCOTT

1836.

**ADVERTISEMENT TO THE THIRD EDITION.**

The present edition has been much enlarged. The author has added a section on the conduct and management of the mother herself, besides several other important amendments and additions. The whole has also been carefully revised, and we cannot but indulge the hope that no popular work of the kind will be found more perfect, or more worthy of the public confidence.

## CONTENTS.

### CHAPTER I. THE NURSERY.

General remarks. Importance of a Nursery—generally overlooked. Its walls—ceiling—windows—chimney. Two apartments. Sliding partition. Reasons for this arrangement. Objections to carpets. Furniture, &c. Feather beds. Holes or crevices. Currents of air. Cats and dogs. "Sucking the child's breath." Brilliant objects. Squinting. Causes of blindness.

## CHAPTER II. TEMPERATURE.

General principle—"Keep cool." Our own sensations not always to be trusted. Thermometer. Why infants require more external heat than adults. Means of warmth. Air heated in other apartments. Clothes taking fire. Stove—railing around it. Excess of heat—its dangers.

## CHAPTER III. VENTILATION.

General ignorance of the constitution of the atmosphere. The subject briefly explained. Oxygen gas. Nitrogen. Carbonic acid. Fires, candles, and breathing dependent on oxygen. Danger from carbonic acid. How it destroys people. Impurity of the air arising from lamps and candles. Other sources of impurity. Experiment of putting the candle under the bed-clothes. Covering the heads of infants while sleeping—its dangers. Proportions of oxygen and nitrogen in pure and impure air. No wonder children become sickly. Particular means of ventilating rooms. Caution in regard to lamps. Washing, ironing, cooking, &c., in a nursery. Their evil tendency. Fumigation—camphor, vinegar.

## CHAPTER IV. THE CHILD'S DRESS.

General principles—1. To cover us; 2. To defend us from cold; 3. from injury.

### SEC. 1. *Swathing the Body*.

Buffon's remarks. Transforming children into mummies. Use of a belly-band. Evils produced by having it too tight. Cripples sometimes made. Absurdity of confining the arms. Infants should be made happy.

### SEC. 2. *Form of the Dress*.

Curious suggestion of a London writer. Advantages of his plan. Killing with kindness. Dr. Buchan's opinion. Conformity to fashion. Tight-lacing the chest. Its effects—dangerous. Physiology of the chest. Its motions. An attempt to make the subject intelligible. Serious mistakes of some writers. Appeal to facts. Color of females. Their breathing. Their diseases. Customs of Tunis. Our own customs little less ridiculous.

### SEC. 3. *Material.*

Flannel in cold weather. Its use—1. As a kind of flesh brush; 2. As a protection against taking cold; 3. As means of equalizing the temperature. Clothing should be kept clean—often changed—color—lightness—softness. Cotton apt to take fire. Silk expensive. Linen not warm enough. Flannel under-clothes.

### SEC. 4. *Quantity.*

The power of habit, in this respect. Opinion that no clothing is necessary. Anecdote of Alexander and the Scythian. Argument from analogy. Begin right, in early life. We generally use too much clothing. Should clothing be often varied? —objections to it. Avoid dampness.

### SEC. 5. *Caps.*

How caps produce disease. Nature's head-dress. Miserable apology for caps. What diseases are avoided by going with the head bare. Judicious remarks of a foreign writer. Covering the "open of the head." Wetting the head with spirits.

### SEC. 6. *HatsandBonnets.*

Hats usually too warm. No covering needed in the house; and but little in the sun or rain. Is it dangerous to go with the head always bare?

### SEC. 7. *CoveringfortheFeet.*

The feet should be well covered. Why. Rule of medical men. No garters. Objections to covering the feet considered. Shoes useful. Not too thick. Thick soles. Mr. Locke's opinion.

### SEC. 8. *Pins.*

These ought not to be used. Why. Substitutes. Practice of Dr. Dewees. Needles— their danger. Shocking anecdote.

### SEC. 9. *RemainingWet.*

Changing wet clothing. Monstrous error—its evils. Clean as well as dry. A lame excuse for negligence. No excuse sufficient but poverty.

### SEC. 10. *RemarksontheDr essofBoys.*

Every restraint of body or limb injurious. Tight jackets. Stiff stocks and thick cravats. Boots. Evils of having them too tight. A painful sight.

### SEC. 11. *On the Dress of Girls.*

Clothing should be loose for girls or boys. Girls to be kept warmer than boys. Few girls comfortable, at home or abroad. Going out of warm rooms into the night air. How it promotes disease.

## CHAPTER V. CLEANLINESS.

Physiology of the human skin. Of checking perspiration. Diseases thus produced. "Dirt" not "healthy." How the mistake originated. "Smell of the earth." Effect of uncleanliness on the morals. Filthiness produces bowel complaints. Changing dress for the sake of cleanliness.

## CHAPTER VI. BATHING.

Practice of savage nations. Rather dangerous. Mistake of Rousseau. Plunging into cold water at birth may produce immediate death. Hundreds injured where one is benefited. Spirits added to the water. First washings of the child—should be thorough. Rules in regard to the temperature of both the water and the air. Washing an introduction to bathing. Hour for bathing changes with age. Temperature of the water. Size of a bathing vessel. Unreasonable fears of the warm bath. How they arose. A list of common whims. Apology for opposing cold baths. Dr Dewees' eight objections to them. Does cold water harden? Cold bath sometimes useful under the care of a skilful physician. Its danger in other cases. Rules for using the cold bath, if used at all. Securing a glow after it. General management. Proper hour. Coming out of the bath. Dressing. Singing. Bathing after a meal. Local bathing. Tea-spoonful of water in the mouth. Its use. The shower bath. Vapor bath. Medicated bath. Sponging. Conveniences for bathing indispensable to every family. General neglect of bathing. Attention of the Romans to this subject. We treat domestic animals better than children.

## CHAPTER VII. FOOD.

### SEC. 1. *General Principles.*

The mother's milk the only appropriate food of infants. Unreasonableness of some mothers. The tendency to ape foreign fashions. Nursing does not weaken the mother.

## SEC. 2. *Conduct of the Mother*.

Much depends on the mother. Opinions of medical societies. Mothers sometimes make children drunkards. The general fondness for excitements. Hints to those whom it concerns. Caution to mothers. Opinions of Dr. Dewees. Slavery of mothers to strong drink and exciting food. Opinions of the Charleston Board of Health.

## SEC. 3. *Nursing, how often*.

Children should never be nursed to quiet them. Stomach must have time for rest. Regular seasons for nursing. Once in three hours. Difference of constitution. Indulgence does not strengthen. Feeble children require the strictest management. Nothing should be given between meals.

## SEC. 4. *Quantity of Food*.

Errors. Repetition of aliment. Variety. Children over-fed. Appetite not a safe guide. Training to gluttony. Illustrations of the principle. Mankind eat twice as much as is necessary.

## SEC. 5. *How long should Milk be the only Food?*

First change in diet. Objections of mothers. Choice bits. Ignorance of the nature of digestion. What digestion is. Food which the author of nature assigned.

## SEC. 6. *On Feeding before Teething*.

When feeding before teething is necessary. Diet of mothers. Substitute for the mother's milk. How prepared. Variety not necessary to the infant. Milk best from the same cow. Vessels in which it is used should be clean. Sweet milk not heated too much. Not frozen. Disgusting practices. Pure water. If not pure, boil it. Best of sugar. Is sugar injurious? When the state of the mother's health forbids nursing. Use of sucking-bottles. Feeding should in all cases be slow. Jolting children after eating. Tossing. Sucking-bottle as a plaything. Evils of using it as such. Dirty vessels. Poisonous ones. Character of nurses. Nursing at both breasts. Age of the nurse. Parents should have the oversight, even of a nurse.

## SEC. 7. *From Teething to Weaning*.

Proper age for weaning. Cullen's opinion. Proper season of the year. When the teeth have fairly protruded. First food given. New forms of food. Animal broth.

## SEC. 8. *During the Process of Weaning*.

The spring the best time for weaning. Should not be too sudden. The process—how managed. Exciting an aversion to the breast. What solid food should first be given. Buchan's opinion. Health of the mother. She should—if possible—avoid medicine.

## SEC. 9. *Food subsequently to Weaning.*

Views of Dr. Cadogan. Half the children that come into the world go out of it before they are good for anything. Why? Owing chiefly to errors in nursing, feeding, and clothing. Simplicity of children's food. Picture of a modern table. Every dish tortured till it is spoiled. Plain, simple food, generally despised. How bread is now regarded. How it ought to be. Mr. Locke's opinion in favor of bread for young children, and against the use of animal food. Does not differ materially from that of most medical writers. Vegetable food generally preferred to animal. What is true of youth, in this respect, is true of every age, with slight exceptions. Who require most food. Mere bread and water not best. Bread the staple article of diet. Best kind of bread. Objections to it. How groundless they are. Fondness, for hot, new bread not natural. Fondness of change. What it indicates. How it is caused. Train up a child in the way he should go. We can like what food we please. Second best kind of bread. Other kinds. Plain puddings. Indian cakes. Salt may be used, in moderate quantity, but no other condiments. Of butter, cheese, milk, &c. Potatoes, turnips, onions, beets, and other roots. Beans, peas, and asparagus. No fat or gravies should be used.

## SEC. 10. *Remarks on Fruit.*

Diversity of opinion. The cholera. Fruits useful. Seven plain rules in regard to them. Other rules. A mistake corrected. Fruit before breakfast. Four arguments in its favor. Particular fruits. Apples. Why fruits brought to market are generally unfit to be eaten. Are good, ripe fruits difficult of digestion? Cooking the apple? A man who lives entirely on apples. Cutting down orchards. Pears, peaches, melons, grapes. Mixing improper substances with summer fruits.

## SEC. 11. *Confectionary.*

Confectionary sometimes poisonous. Case in New York. All, or nearly all confectionaries injurious. Physical evils attending their use. Intellectual evils. Moral evils. The last most to be dreaded. Slaves to confectionary are on the road to gluttony, drunkenness, or debauchery—perhaps all three.

## SEC. 12. *Pastry.*

Dr. Paris's opinion of pastry. Various forms of it. Hot flour bread a species of it. Produces, among other evils, eruptions on the face. Appeal to mothers.

## SEC. 13. *Crude, or Raw Substances.*

Salads, herbs, &c.—raw—cooked. Nuts, spices, mustard, horseradish, onions, cucumbers, pickles, &c. None of these should be used, except as medicine.

# CHAPTER VIII. DRINKS.

Infants need little drink. Adults, even, generally drink to cool themselves. Simple water the best drink. Opinions of Dr. Oliver and Dr. Dewees. Animal food increases thirst. Only one real drink in the world. The true object of all drink. Tea, coffee, chocolate, beer, &c. Milk and water, molasses and water, &c. Cider, wine, and ardent spirits. Bad food and drink the most prolific sources of disease. Children naturally prefer water. Danger of hot drinks. Cold drinks. Mischiefs they produce. Caution to mothers. Extracts. Drinking cold water, while hot.

## CHAPTER IX. GIVING MEDICINE.

"Prevention" better than "cure." Nine in ten infantile diseases caused by errors in diet and drink. Signs of failing health. Causes of a bad breath. Flesh eaters. Gormandizers. General rule for preventing disease. When to call a physician.

## CHAPTER X. EXERCISE.

### SEC. 1. *RockingintheCradle.*

Objections to the use of cradles. Under what circumstances they are least objectionable.

### SEC. 2. *CarryingintheArms.*

Carrying in the arms a suitable exercise for the first two months of life. Danger of too early sitting up. Improper position in the arms. Mothers must see to this themselves. Motion in the arms should be gentle. No tossing, running, or jumping. Infants should not always be carried on the same arm.

### SEC. 3. *Creeping.*

Creeping useful to health. Why. Go-carts and leading strings prohibited. The longer children creep, the better. Their progress in learning to stand. Let it be slow and natural. Let it be, as much as possible, by their own voluntary efforts.

### SEC. 4. *Walking.*

Walking in the nursery. Walking abroad. Hoisting children into carriages. Walks should not become fatiguing.

### SEC. 5. *RidinginCarriages.*

Carriages useful before children can walk. Their construction. Should be drawn steadily. Position of the child in them: Falling asleep. How long this exercise should be continued.

### SEC. 6. *Riding on Horseback.*

Never safe for infants. Riding schools. Objections to riding on horseback, while very young. Tends to cruelty and tyranny.

## CHAPTER XI. AMUSEMENTS.

Universal need of amusements. Why so necessary. Error of schools. Error of families. Infant schools, as often conducted, particularly injurious. Lessons, or tasks, should be short. Mistakes of some manual labor schools. Of particular amusements in the nursery. With small wooden cubes—pictures—shuttlecock—the rocking horse—tops and marbles—backgammon—checkers—morrice—dice—nine-pins—skipping the rope—trundling the hoop—playing at ball—kites—skating and swimming—dissected maps—black boards—elements of letters—dissected pictures.

## CHAPTER XII. CRYING.

Its importance. Danger of repressing a tendency to cry. Anecdote from Dr. Rush. Physiology of crying. Folly of attempting wholly to suppress it.

## CHAPTER XIII. LAUGHING.

"Laugh and be fat." Laughing is healthy. A common error. Monastic notions yet too prevalent on this subject.

## CHAPTER XIV. SLEEP.

General remarks. A prevalent mistake. A hint to fathers. Few Catos. Everything left to mothers.

## SEC. 1. *Hour for Repose.*

Night the season of repose, generally. Infants require all hours. Sleeping in dark rooms. Excess of caution. Habit of sleeping amid noise.

## SEC. 2. *Place.*

Where the infant should sleep. Why alone. Poisoning by impure air. Illustration. Proofs. Friedlander. Dr. Dewees. Destruction of children by mothers. Anecdote. Moral reasons for having children sleep alone. Sleeping with the aged. Sleeping with cats and dogs.

## SEC. 3 *Purity of the Air*.

Nurseries. Windows open during the night. Lowering them from the top. Habit of Dr. Gregory. Going abroad in the open air.

## SEC. 4. *The Bed.*

No feathers should be used. They are too warm. Their effluvia oppressive. Other objections to their use. Mattresses. Air beds. Beds of cut straw. Soft beds. Testimony of physicians. The pillow. Dampness. Curtains. Warming the bed. Beds recently occupied by the sick.

## SEC. 5. *The Covering.*

Light covering. Mistakes of some mothers. Covering the head with bed clothes.

## SEC. 6. *Night Dresses.*

As little dress during sleep as possible. No caps. No stockings. Loose night shirt. No tight articles of nightdress. Frequent exchanging of clothes.

## SEC. 7. *Posture of the Body*.

Sleeping on the back—on the sides. Position of the head. The infant's bedstead. Sir Charles Bell. Darkening the room.

## SEC. 8. *State of the Mind.*

Mental quiet favorable to sleep. Crying to sleep. A good father. All anxiety should be avoided.

## SEC. 9. *Quality of Sleep.*

Soundness of our sleep. Nightmare. How produced. Late reading. Late suppers. Influence of religion on sleep. Different opinions about sleep. Truth midway between extremes. Effect of silence and darkness on our sleep. Of sleep before midnight. Light unfavorable to sleep.

### SEC. 10. *Quantity.*

Infants need to sleep nearly the whole time. Number of hours required for sleep. Opinions of eminent men. The author's own opinion. Statements of Macnish. Estimates on the loss of time by over-sleeping. Hint to young mothers.

## CHAPTER XV. EARLY RISING.

All children naturally early risers. Evils of sitting up late at night. Excitements in the evening. The morning, by its beauties, invites us abroad. Example of parents. Forbidding children to rise early. Keeping them out of the way. Burning them up. "Lecturing" them. What is an early hour?

## CHAPTER XVI. HARDENING THE CONSTITUTION.

Mistakes about hardening children. Their clothing. Much cold enfeebles. The Scotch Highlanders. The two extremes equally fatal—over-tenderness and neglect. An interesting anecdote from Dr. Dewees.

## CHAPTER XVII. SOCIETY.

Duty of mothers in this matter. Children prefer the society of parents. Importance of other society. Necessity of society. Early diffidence. Selecting companions. Moral effects of society on the young. Parents should play with their children.

## CHAPTER XVIII. EMPLOYMENTS.

Influence of mothers over daughters. Anecdote of Benjamin West. Anecdote of a poor mother. Of set lessons and lectures. Daughters under the mother's eye. Disliking domestic employments. Miserable housewives—not to be wondered at. Mistake of one class of men. Mr. Flint's opinion.

# CHAPTER XIX. EDUCATION OF THE SENSES.

Extent to which the senses can be improved. Case of the blind. The Indians. Julia Brace. Tailors, painters, &c.

## SEC. 1. *Hearing.*

Injury done by caps. Syringing the ears. Anecdote of deafness from neglect. Means of improving the hearing.

## SEC. 2. *Seeing.*

Importance of seeing. Near-sighted people—why so common. Heat of our rooms. Very fine print. Spectacles. Reading when tired. Rubbing the eyes. Cold water to the eyes.

## SEC. 3. *TastingandSmelling.*

Benumbing the senses. How this has often been done. The teeth. How to preserve them.

## SEC. 4. *Feeling.*

Corpulence and slovenliness. Sense of touch. The blind—how taught to read. Hint to parents. The hand. Neglecting the left hand. Physiology of the hand and arm. Evils of being able to use but one hand. Both should be educated.

# CHAPTER XX. ABUSES.

Bad seats for children at table and elsewhere. Why children hate Sunday. Seats at Sabbath school—at church—at district schools. Suspending children between the heavens and the earth. Cushions to sit on. Seats with backs. Children in factories. Evils produced. Bodily punishment. Striking the heads of children very injurious. Beating across the middle of the body. Anecdote of a teacher. Concluding advice to mothers.

---

# PREFACE.

There is a prejudice abroad, to some extent, against agitating the questions—"What shall we eat? What shall we drink? and Wherewithal shall we be clothed?"—not so much because the Scriptures have charged us not to be over "anxious" on the subject, as because those who pay the least attention to what they eat and drink, are supposed to be, after all, the most healthy.

It is not difficult to ascertain how this opinion originated. There are a few individuals who are perpetually thinking and talking on this subject, and who would fain comply with appropriate rules, if they knew what they were, and if a certain definite course, pursued a few days only, would change their whole condition, and completely restore a shattered or ruined constitution. But their ignorance of the laws which govern the human frame, both in sickness and in health, and their indisposition to pursue any proposed plan for their improvement long enough to receive much permanent benefit from it, keep them, notwithstanding all they say or do, always deteriorating.

Then, on the other hand, there are a few who, in consequence of possessing by nature very strong constitutions, and laboring at some active and peculiarly healthy employment, are able for a few, and perhaps even for many years, to set all the rules of health at defiance.

Now, strange as it may seem, these cases, though they are only exceptions (and those more apparent than real) to the general rule, are always dwelt upon, by those who are determined to live as they please, and to put no restraint either upon themselves or their appetites. For nothing can be plainer—so it seems to me—than that, taking mankind by families, or what is still better, by larger portions, they are most free from pain and disease, as well as most healthy and happy, who pay the most attention to the laws of human health, that is, those laws or rules by whose observance alone, that health can be certainly and permanently secured.

But these families and communities are most healthy and happy, not because they live in a proper manner, by fits and starts, but because they have, from some cause or other, adopted and persevered in HABITS which, compared with the habits of other families, or other communities, are preferable; that is, more in obedience to the laws which govern the human constitution. Not that even *they* are "without sin" or error on this subject—gross error too—but because their errors are fewer or less destructive than those of their neighbors.

Now is it possible that any intelligent father or mother of a family, whose diet, clothing, exercise, &c. are thus comparatively well regulated, would derive no benefit from the perusal of works which treat candidly, rationally, and dispassionately, on these points? Is there a mother in the community who is so destitute of reason and common sense as not to desire the light of a broader experience in regard to the tendency of things than she has had, or possibly can have, in her own family? Is there one who will not be aided by understanding not only that a certain thing or course is better than another, but also WHY it is so?

It is by no means the object of this little work to set people to watching their stomachs from meal to meal, in regard to the effects of food, drink, &c.; for nothing in the world is better calculated to make dyspeptics than this. It is true, indeed, that some things may be obviously and greatly injurious, taken only once; and when they are so, they should be avoided. But in general, it is the effect of a habitual use of certain things for a long time together—and the longer the experiment the better—which we are to observe.

A book to guide mothers in the formation of early good habits in their offspring, should be the result of long observation and much experiment on these points, but more especially of a thorough understanding of human physiology. It should not consist so much of the conceits of a single brain—perhaps half turned—as of the logical deductions of severe science, and facts gleaned from the world's history.

Here is a nation, or tribe of men, bringing up children to certain habits, from generation to generation—and such and such is their character. Here, again, is another large portion of our race, who, under similar circumstances of climate, &c. &c., have, for several hundred years, educated their children very differently, and with different results. A comparison of things on a large scale, together with a close attention to the constitution and relations of the human system, affords ground for drawing conclusions which are or may be useful. If this book shall not afford light derived from such sources, it were far better that it had never been written. If it only sets people to watching over the effects of things taken or used only for a single day, instead of leading them from early infancy to form in their children such habits as will preclude, in a great measure, the necessity of watching ourselves daily, then let the day perish from the memory of the writer, in which the plan of bringing it forth to the world was conceived. But he is confident of better things. He does not believe that a work which, to such an extent, GIVES THE REASON WHY, will be productive of more evil than good. On the contrary, it must, if read, have the opposite effect.

I do not deny that even after the formation of the best habits, there will be a necessity of paying some attention to what we eat and what we drink, from day to day, and from hour to hour; but only that the tendency of this work is not to increase this necessity, but on the contrary, to diminish it. In my own view; these occasions of inquiry in regard to what is right, *physically* as well as *morally*, are one part of our trials in this world—one means of forming our characters. We are constantly tempted to excess and to error, in spite of the most firm habits of self-denial which can be formed. If we resist temptation, our characters are improved. And it is by self-denial and self-government in these smaller matters, that we are to hope for nearly all the progress we can ever make in the great work of self-education. Great trials of character come but seldom; and when they come, we are often armed against them; but these little trials and temptations, coming upon us every hour—these it is, after all, that give shape to our characters, and make us constantly growing either better or worse, both in the sight of God and man. But, as I have repeatedly said, the object of this work is to diminish rather than to increase the frequency of these trials, useful though they may be, if duly improved, in the formation of virtuous, and even of holy character.

There is a sense in which every infant may be said to be born healthy, so that we may not only adopt the language of the poet, Bowring, and say

—"a child is born;
Take it, and make it a bud of *moral* beauty,"

but we may also add—Take it and make it beautiful *physically*. For though a hereditary predisposition undoubtedly renders some individuals more susceptible than others to particular diseases, yet when the bodily organization of an infant is complete, and the degree of vitality which nature gives it is sufficient to propel the machinery of the frame, it can scarcely be regarded as in any other state than that of health.

Now if it be the intention of divine Providence (and who will doubt that it is?) that the animal body should be capable of resisting with impunity the impressions of heat, cold, light, air, and the various external influences to which, at birth, it is subjected, it may be properly asked why this primitive state of health cannot be maintained, and diseases, and medicines, and even PREVENTIVES wholly avoided.

But the reason is obvious. Civilized society has placed the human race in artificial circumstances. Instead of listening to the dictates of reason, making ourselves acquainted with the nature of the human constitution, and studying to preserve it in health and vigor, we yield to the government of ignorance and presumption. The first moment, even, in which we draw breath, sees us placed under the control of individuals who are totally inadequate to the important charge of preserving the infant constitution in its original state, and aiding its progress to maturity. And thus it is that though infants, as a general rule, may be said to be born healthy, few actually remain so. Seldom, indeed, do we find a person who has arrived at maturity wholly free from disease, even in those parts of our country which are reckoned to have the most healthy climate.

It is indeed commonly said, that a large proportion, both of children and adults, among the agricultural portion of our population, are healthy. But it is not so. There is room for doubt whether, on the whole, the farmers of this country are healthier than the mechanics, or much more so than the manufacturers; or the whole mass of the country population healthier than that of the crowded city. The causes of disease are sufficiently numerous, in all places and conditions; and this will continue to be the fact, not merely until parents and teachers shall become more enlightened, but until many generations have been trained under their enlightened influence.

If the children and adults among our agricultural population derive from their employments in the open air a more ruddy appearance than those either of the city or country who are confined more to their rooms; or to a vitiated atmosphere, and to numerous other sources of disease, and if they *appear* more favored with health, I have learned, by accurate observation, that these appearances are somewhat deceptive. Their active sports and employments in the open air give them a stronger appetite than any other class of people; and the indulgence of this appetite, not only with articles which are heating or indigestible in their nature, but with an unreasonable quantity even of those which are considered highly proper, is almost in an exact proportion. And it is hence scarcely possible for the causes of disease and premature death to be more operative in factories and in cities than in farm houses and the country. Indeed it may be questioned whether the abuses of the ANIMAL part of man—more common in some of their forms in country than in city—though they may be less conspicuous, are not more certainly and even more immediately destructive than those abuses which, in city life, and bustle, and competition, affect more the MORAL nature.

Be that as it may, however—for this is not the place for the grave discussion of so broad a question—one thing, to my mind, is perfectly clear, namely, that until physical education shall receive more attention from all those who hold the sacred office of instructors of the young, humanity can neither be much elevated nor improved. Mothers and schoolmasters especially—they who, as Dr. Rush says, plant the seeds of nearly all the good or evil in the world—must understand, most deeply and thoroughly, the laws which regulate the various provinces of the little world in which the soul resides, and which, like so many states of a great confederacy, have not only their separate interests and rights, but certain common and general ones; as well as those laws by which the human constitution is related to and connected with the objects which everywhere surround, and influence, and limit, and extend it.

This book contains little, if anything, new to those who are already familiar with anatomy and physiology. Indeed, whatever may be its claims, its merits or its demerits, it disclaims novelty. It is, indeed, in one point of view, *original*;—I mean in its form, manner, and arrangement. What I have written is chiefly from my own resources—the results of patient study and observation, and careful reflection; but that study and observation of human nature, and this reflection, have been greatly aided by reading the writings of others.

In the prosecution of the task which I had assigned myself, no work has been of more service to me than an octavo volume of 548 pages, by Dr. Wm. P. Dewees, of Philadelphia, entitled, "A Treatise on the Physical and Medical Treatment of Children." It is one of the most valuable works on Physical Education in the English language, as is evident from the fact that notwithstanding its expense—three or four dollars—it has, in nine years, gone through five editions. If it were written in such a style, and published at such a price as would bring it within reach of the minds and purses of the mass of the community, its sale would have been, I think, much greater still; and the good which it has accomplished would have been increased tenfold.

If the "YOUNG MOTHER" should be favorably received by the American community, and prove extensively useful, it will undoubtedly be owing to the fact that it presents so large a collection of facts and principles on the great subject of physical education, in a manner so practical, and at a price which is very low. To accomplish an object so desirable is by no means an easy task. It was once said by the author of a huge volume, that he wrote so large a work because he had not time to prepare a smaller one. And however unaccountable it may be to those who have not made the trial, it may be safely asserted, that to present, within limits so small, anything like a system of Physical Education for the guidance of young mothers, requires much more time, and labor, and patience, than to prepare a work on the same subject twice as large.

Nor is it to be expected, after all, that the work is, in all respects, perfect. I have indeed done what I could to render it so; but am conscious that future inquiries may lead to the discovery of errors. Should such discoveries be made, they will be cheerfully acknowledged and corrected; truth being, as it should be, the leading object.

# CHAPTER I.

## THE NURSERY.

*General remarks. Importance of a Nursery—generally overlooked. Its walls—ceiling—windows—chimney. Two apartments. Sliding partition. Reasons for this arrangement. Objections to carpets. Furniture, &c. Feather beds. Holes or crevices. Currents of air. Cats and dogs. "Sucking the child's breath." Brilliant objects. Squinting. Causes of blindness.*

It is far from being in the power of every young mother to procure a suitable room for a nursery. In the present state of society, the majority must be contented with such places as they can get. Still there are various reasons for saying what a nursery should be. 1. It may be of service to those who *have* the power of selection. 2. Information cannot injure those who *have not*. 3. It may lead those who have wealth to extend the hand of charity in this important direction; for there are not a few who have little sympathy with the wants and distresses of the adult poor, who will yet open their hearts and unfold their hands for the relief of suffering *infancy*.

Among those who have what is called a nursery, few select for this purpose the most appropriate part of the building. It is not unfrequently the one that can best be spared, is most retired, or most convenient. Whether it is most favorable to the health and happiness of its occupants, is usually at best a secondary consideration.

But this ought not so to be. A nursery should never, for example, be on a ground floor, or in a shaded situation, or in any circumstances which expose it to dampness, or hinder the occasional approach of the light of the sun. It should be spacious, with dry walls, high ceiling, and tight windows. The latter should always be so constructed that the upper sash can be lowered when we wish to admit or exclude air. It should have a chimney, if possible; but if not, there should be suitable holes in the ceiling, for the purposes of ventilation.

The windows should have shutters, so that the room, when necessary, can be darkened—and green curtains. Some writers say that the windows should have cross bars before them; but if they do not descend within three feet of the floor, such an arrangement can hardly be required.

It is highly desirable that every nursery should consist of two rooms, opening into each other; or what is still better, of one large room, with a sliding or swinging partition in the middle. The use of this is, that the mother and child may retire to one, while the other is being swept or ventilated. They would thus avoid damp air, currents, and dust. Such an arrangement would also give the occupants a room, fresh, clean and sweet, in the morning, (which is a very great advantage,) after having rendered the air of the other foul by sleeping in it.

In winter, and while there is an infant in the nursery, just beginning to walk, it is recommended by many to cover the floor with a carpet. The only advantage which they mention is, that it secures the child from injury if it falls. But I have seldom seen lasting injury inflicted by simple falls on the hard floor; and there are so many objections to carpeting a nursery, since it favors an accumulation of dust, bad air, damp, grease, and other impurities, that it seems to me preferable to omit it. Many physicians, I must own, recommend carpets during winter, though not in summer; and in no case, unless they are well shaken and aired, at least once a week.

No furniture should be admissible, except the beds for the mother and child, a table, and a few chairs. With the best writers and highest authorities on the subject, I am decidedly of opinion that all feather beds ought effectually and forever to be excluded from nurseries. The reasons for this prohibition will appear hereafter.

Every nursery should, if possible, be free from holes or crevices; otherwise the occupants will be exposed to currents of air, and their sometimes terrible and always injurious consequences. The room may, in this way, be kept at a lower medium temperature—a point of very great importance.

Cats and dogs, I believe, are usually excluded from the nursery; if not, they ought to be. For though the apprehension of cats "sucking the child's breath," is wholly groundless, yet they may be provoked by the rude attacks of a child to inflict upon it a lasting injury. Besides, they assist, by respiration, in contaminating the air, like all other animals.

If there are, in the nursery, objects which, from the vivacity or brilliancy of their colors, attract the attention of the child, they should never be presented to them sideways, or immediately over their heads. The reason for this caution is, that children seek, and pursue almost instinctively, bright objects; and are thus liable to contract a habit of moving their eyes in an oblique direction, which *may* terminate in squinting.

Many parents seem to take great pleasure in indulging the young infant in looking at these bright objects; especially a lamp or a candle. If the child is naturally strong and vigorous, no immediate perceptible injury may arise; but I am confident in the opinion that the result is often quite otherwise. For many weeks, if not many months of their early existence, they should not be permitted to sit or lie and gaze at any bright object, be it ever so weak or distant, unless placed exactly before their eyes; and even in the latter case, it were better to avoid it.

Heat is also injurious to the eyes of all, and of course not less so to children than to adults. But when a strong light and heat are conjoined, as is the case of sitting around a large blazing fire—the former custom of New England—it is no wonder if the infantile eyes become early injured. No wonder that the generation now on the stage, early subjected to these abuses, should be found almost universally in the use of spectacles.

This may be the most proper place for observing that great care ought to be taken, at the birth of the child, to prevent a too sudden exposure of the tender organ of vision to the light. We believe this caution is generally omitted by the American physician, though it is one which accords with the plainest dictates of common sense. Who of us has not experienced the pain of emerging suddenly from the darkness of a cellar to the ordinary light of day? The strongest eyes of the adult are scarcely able to bear the transition. How much more painful to the tender organs of the new-born infant must be the change to which it is so frequently subjected? And how easy it is to prevent the pain and danger of the change, by more effectually darkening the room into which it is introduced!

# CHAPTER II.

## TEMPERATURE.

*General principle—"Keep cool." Our own sensations not always to be trusted. Thermometer. Why infants require more external heat than adults. Means of warmth. Air heated in other apartments. Clothes taking fire. Stove—railing around it. Excess of heat—its dangers.*

There is one general principle, on this subject, which is alike applicable to all persons and circumstances. It is, to keep a little too cool, rather than in the slightest degree too warm. In other words, the lowest temperature which is compatible with comfort, is, in all cases, best adapted to health; and a slight degree of coldness, provided it amount not to a chill, and is not long continued, is more safe than the smallest unnecessary degree of warmth.

But the application of this rule to those over whom we have control, is not without its difficulties. Our own sensations are so variable, independently of external and obvious causes, that we cannot at all times judge for others, especially for infants. The absolute and real state of temperature in a room can only be ascertained by the aid of a thermometer; and no nursery should ever be without one. It should be placed, however, in such a situation as to indicate the real temperature of the atmosphere, and not where it will give a false result.

No mother should forget that the infant, at birth, has not the power of generating heat, internally, to the extent which it possesses afterward. The lungs have as yet but a feeble, inefficient action. The purification of the blood, through their agency, is not only incomplete, but the heat evolved is as yet inconsiderable. In the absence of internal heat, then, there is an increased demand externally. If 60° be deemed suitable for most other persons, the new-born infant may, for a few days, require 65° or even 70°.

Much may and should be done in preserving the child in a proper temperature by means of its clothing. On this point I shall speak at length, in another part of this work. My present purpose is simply to treat of the temperature of the nursery.

The best way of warming a nursery—or indeed any other room, where MERE warmth is demanded—is by means of air heated in other apartments, and admitted through openings in the floor or fire-place. The air is not only thus made more pure, but every possibility of accidents, such as having the clothes take fire, is precluded. This last consideration is one of very great importance, and I hope will not be much longer overlooked in infantile education.

Next to that, in point of usefulness and safety, is a stove, placed near or IN the fire-place, and defended by an iron railing. Most people prefer an open stove; and on some accounts it is indeed preferable, especially where it is desirable to burn coal. Still I think that the direct rays of the heat, and the glare of light from open stoves and fire-places, particularly for the young, form a very serious objection to their use.

One of the strongest objections to open stoves and fire-places in the nursery is, the increased exposure to accidents. I know it is said that this evil may be avoided by laying aside the use of cotton, and wearing nothing but worsted or flannel. This is indeed true; but I do not like the idea of being compelled to dress children in flannel or worsted, at all times when the least particle of fire is demanded; for this would be to wear this stimulating kind of clothing, in our climate, the greater part of the year.

Besides, I write for many mothers who are compelled to use cotton, on account of the expense of flannel. And if the stove be a close one, and well defended by a railing, cotton will seldom expose to danger. Still, as has been already said, the introduction of heated air from another apartment, whenever it can possibly be afforded, is incomparably better than either stoves or fire-places.

Dr. Dewees is fully persuaded that the excessive heat of nurseries has occasioned a great mortality among very young children. "In the first place," he says, "it over-stimulates them; and in the second, it renders them so susceptible of cold, that any draught of cold air endangers their lives. They are in a constant perspiration, which is frequently checked by an exposure to even an atmosphere of moderate temperature."

# CHAPTER III.

## VENTILATION.

General ignorance of the constitution of the atmosphere. The subject briefly explained. Oxygen gas. Nitrogen. Carbonic acid. Fires, candles, and breathing dependent on oxygen. Danger from carbonic acid. How it destroys people. Impurity of the air by means of lamps and candles. Other sources of impurity. Experiment of putting the candle under the bed-clothes. Covering the heads of infants while sleeping—its dangers. Proportions of oxygen and nitrogen in pure and impure air. No wonder children become sickly. Particular means of ventilating rooms. Caution in regard to lamps. Washing, ironing, cooking, &c., in a nursery. Their evil tendency. Fumigation—camphor, vinegar.

Few people take sufficient pains to preserve the air in any of their apartments pure; for few know what the constitution of our atmosphere is, and in how many ways and with what ease it is rendered impure.

It is not my purpose to go into a learned, scientific account in this place, or even in this work, of the constitution of the atmosphere. A few plain statements are all that are indispensable. The atmosphere which we breathe is composed of two different airs or gases. One of these is called oxygen, [Footnote: Oxygen gas is the chief supporter of combustion, as well as of respiration. It is the vital part, as it were, of the air. No animal or vegetable could long exist without it. And yet if alone, unmixed, it is too pure and too refined for animals to breathe. Nitrogen gas, on the contrary, while alone, will not support either respiration or combustion; mixed, however, with oxygen, it dilutes it, and in the most happy manner fits it for reception into the lungs.] and the other nitrogen. There is another gas usually found with these two, in smaller quantity, called carbonic acid gas; but whether it is necessary, in a very small quantity, to health, chemists, I believe, are not agreed. One thing, however, is certain—that if any portion of it is healthful, it must be very little—not more, certainly, than one-fiftieth or one-hundredth of the whole mass.

It is by means of the oxygen it contains, that air sustains life and combustion. Were it not for this, neither fires nor candles would burn, and no animal could breathe a single moment. Breathing consumes this oxygen of the air very rapidly. When the oxygen is present in about a certain proportion, combustion and respiration go on well, but when its natural proportion is diminished, the fire does not burn so well, neither does the candle; and no one can breathe so freely.

Not only are breathing and combustion impeded or disturbed by the diminution of oxygen in the atmosphere, but just in proportion as oxygen is diminished by these two processes, or either of them, carbonic acid is formed, which is not only bad for combustion, but much worse for health. If any considerable quantity of it is inhaled, it appears to be an absolute poison to the human system; and if in *very large quantity*, will often cause immediate death.

It is this gas, accumulated in large quantities, that destroys so many people in close rooms, where there is no chimney, nor any other place for the bad air to escape. But it not only kills people outright—it partly kills, that is, it poisons, more or less, hundreds of thousands.

In a nursery there is the mother and child, and perhaps the nurse, to render the air impure by breathing, the fire and the lamp or candle to contribute to the same result, besides several other causes not yet mentioned. One of these is nearly related to the former. I allude to the fact that our skins, by perspiration and by other means, are a source of much impurity to the atmosphere; a fact which will be more fully explained and illustrated in the chapter on Bathing and Cleanliness. It is only necessary to say, in this place, that it is not the matter of perspiration alone which, issuing from the skin, renders the air impure; there are other exhalations more or less constantly going off from every living body, especially from the lungs; and carbonic acid gas is even formed all over the surface of the skin, as well as by means of the lungs.

One needs no better proof that carbonic acid is formed on the surface of the body, than the fact that after the body has been closely covered all night, if you introduce a candle under the bed-clothes into this confined air, it will be quickly extinguished, because there is too much carbonic acid gas there, and too little oxygen.

We may hence see at once the evil of covering the heads of infants when they lie down—a very common practice. The air, when pure, contains a little more than 20 parts of oxygen, and a little less than 80 of nitrogen. Breathing this air, as I have already shown, consumes the oxygen, which is so necessary to life and health, and leaves in its place an increase of nitrogen and carbonic acid gas, which are not necessary to health, and the latter of which is even positively injurious. But when the oxygen, instead of forming 20 or more parts in 100 of the atmosphere of the nursery, is reduced to 15 or 18 parts only, and the carbonic acid gas is increased from 1 or 2 parts in 100, to 5, 6, 8 or 10—when to this is added the other noxious exhalations from the body, and from the lamp or candle, fire-place, feather bed, stagnant fluids in the room, &c., &c.—is it any wonder that children, in the end, become sickly? What else could be expected but that the seeds of disease, thus early sown, should in due time spring up, and produce their appropriate fruits?

It is sometimes said that fire in a room purifies it. It undoubtedly does so, to a certain extent, if fresh air be often admitted; but not otherwise.

I have classed feather beds among the common causes of impurity. Dr. Dewees also condemns them, most decidedly; and gives substantial reasons for "driving them out of the nursery."

In speaking of the structure of the room used for a nursery, I have adverted to the importance of having a large or double room, with sliding doors between, in order that the occupants may go into one of them, while the other is being ventilated. But whatever may be the structure of the room, the circumstances of the occupants, or the state of the weather, every nursery ought to be most thoroughly ventilated, once a day, at least; and when the weather is tolerable, twice a day. If there is but one apartment, and fear is entertained of the dampness of the fresh air introduced, or of currents, and if the mother and babe cannot retire, there is a last resort, which is for them to get into bed, and cover themselves a short time with the clothing. For though I have prohibited the covering of the face with the bed-clothes for any considerable length of time together, yet to do so for some fifteen or twenty minutes is an evil of far less magnitude than to suffer an apartment to remain without being ventilated, for twenty-four hours together—a very common occurrence.

When a lamp is kept burning in a nursery during the night, it should always be placed at the door of the stove, or in the chimney place, that its smoke, and the bad airs or gases which are formed, may escape. But it is better, in general, to avoid burning lamps or candles during the night. By means of common matches, a light may be produced, when necessary, almost instantly; especially if you have a spirit lamp in the nursery, or what is still better, one of spirit gas—that is, a mixture of alcohol and turpentine.

It is highly desirable that all washing, ironing, and cooking should be avoided in the nursery. They load the air with noxious effluvia or vapor, or with particles of dust; none of which ought ever to enter the delicate lungs of an infant.

Fumigations with camphor, vinegar, and other similar substances, have long been in reputation as a means of purifying the air in sick-rooms and nurseries; but they are of very little consequence. Fresh air, if it can be had, is always better.

# CHAPTER IV.

## THE CHILD'S DRESS

General principles. SEC. 1. Swathing the body—its numerous evils.—SEC. 2. Form of the dress. Fashion. Tight lacing—its dangers. Structure and motion of the chest. Diseases from tight lacing.—SEC. 3. Material of dress. Flannel—its uses. Cleanliness. Cotton—silk—linen.—SEC. 4. Quantity of dress. Power of habit. Anecdote. Begin right. Change. Dampness.—SEC. 5. Caps—their evils. Going bare-headed.—SEC. 6. Hats and bonnets.—SEC. 7. Covering for the feet. Stockings. Garters. Shoes—thick soles.—SEC. 8. Pins—their danger. Shocking anecdote.—SEC. 9. Remaining wet.—SEC. 10. Dress of boys. Tight jackets. Stocks and cravats. Boots.—SEC. 11. Dress of girls—should be loose. Temperature. Exposure to the night air.

Dress serves three important purposes:—1. To cover us; 2. To defend us against cold; 3. To defend our bodies and limbs from injury. There is one more purpose of dress; in case of deformity, it seems to improve the appearance.

In all our arrangements in regard to dress, whether of children or of adults, we should ever keep in mind the above principles. The form, fashion, material, application, and quantity of all clothing, especially for infants, ought to be regulated by these three or four rules.

The subject of this chapter is one of so much importance, and embraces such a variety of items, that it will be more convenient, both to the reader and myself, to consider it under several minor heads.

### SEC. 1. *Swathing the Body.*

Buffon, in his "Natural History," says that in France, an infant has hardly enjoyed the liberty of moving and stretching its limbs, before it is put into confinement. "It is swathed," says he, "its head is fixed, its legs are stretched out at full length, and its arms placed straight down by the side of its body. In this manner it is bound tight with cloths and bandages, so that it cannot stir a limb; indeed it is fortunate that the poor thing is not muffled up so as to be unable to breathe."

All swathing, except with a single bandage around the abdomen, is decidedly unreasonable, injurious and cruel. I do not pretend that the remarks of M. Buffon are fully applicable to the condition of infants in the United States. The good sense of the community nowhere permits us to transform a beautiful babe quite into an Egyptian mummy. Still there are many considerable errors on the subject of infantile dress, which, in the progress of my remarks, I shall find it necessary to expose.

The use of a simple band cannot be objected to. It affords a general support to the abdomen, and a particular one to the *umbilicus*. The last point is one of great importance, where there is any tendency to a rupture at this part of the body—a tendency which very often exists in feeble children. And without some support of this kind, crying, coughing, sneezing, and straining in any way, might greatly aggravate the evil, if not produce serious consequences.

But, in order to afford a support to the abdomen in the best manner, it is by no means necessary that the bandage should be drawn very tight. Two thirds of the nurses in this country greatly err in this respect, and suppose that the more tightly a bandage is drawn, the better. It should be firm, but yet gently yielding; and therefore a piece of flannel cut "bias," as it is termed, or, obliquely with respect to the threads of which it is composed, is the most appropriate material.

If the attention of the mother were necessary nowhere else, it would be indispensable in the application of this article. If she do not take special pains to prevent it, the erring though well meaning nurse may so compress the body with the bandage as to produce pain and uneasiness, and sometimes severe colic. Nay, worse evils than even this have been known to arise. When a child sneezes, or coughs, or cries, the abdomen should naturally yield gently; but if it is so confined that it cannot yield where the band is applied, it will yield in an unnatural proportion below, to the great danger of producing a species of rupture, no less troublesome than the one which such tight swathing is designed to prevent.

But besides the bandage already mentioned, no other restraint of the body and limbs of a child is at all admissible. The Creator has kindly ordained that the human body and limbs, and especially its muscles, or moving powers, shall be developed by exercise. Confine an arm or a leg, even in a child of ten years of age, and the limb will not increase either in strength or size as it otherwise would, because its muscles are not exercised; and the fact is still more obvious in infancy.

There is a still deeper evil. On all the limbs are fixed two sets of muscles; one to extend, the other to draw up or bend the limb. If you keep a limb extended for a considerable time, you weaken the one set of muscles; if you keep it bent, you weaken the other. This weakness may become so great that the limb will be rendered useless. There are cases on record—well authenticated—where children, by being obliged to sit in one place on a hard floor, have been made cripples for life. Hundreds of others are injured, though they may not become absolutely crippled.

I repeat it, therefore, their dress should be so free and loose that they may use their little limbs, their neck and their bodies, as much as they please; and in every desired direction. The practices of confining their arms while they lie down, for fear they should scratch themselves with their nails, and of pinning the clothes round their feet, are therefore highly reprehensible. Better that they should even occasionally scratch themselves with their nails, than that they should be made the victims of injurious restraint. Who would think of tying up or muffling the young lamb or kid? And even the young plant—what think you would be the effect, if its leaves and branches could not move gently with the soft breezes? Would the fluids circulate, and health be promoted: or would they stagnate, and a morbid, sickly and dwarfish state be the consequence?

Those whose object is to make infancy, as well as any other period of existence, a season of happiness, will not fail to find an additional motive for giving the little stranger entire freedom in the land whither he has so recently arrived, especially when he seems to enjoy it so much. Who can be so hardened as to confine him, unless compelled by the most pressing necessity?

### SEC. 2. *Form of the Dress.*

On this subject a writer in the London Literary Gazette of some eight or ten years ago, lays down the following general directions, to which, in cold weather, there can be but one possible objection, which is, they are not *alamode,* and are not, therefore, likely to be followed.

"All that a child requires, so far as regards clothing, in the first month of its existence, is a simple covering for the trunk and extremities of the body, made of a material soft and agreeable to the skin, and which can retain, in an equable degree, the animal temperature. These qualities are to be found in perfection in fine flannel; and I recommend that the only clothing, for the first month or six weeks, be a square piece of flannel, large enough to involve fully and overlap the whole of the babe, with the exception of the head, which should be left totally uncovered. This wrapper should be fixed by a button near the breast, and left so loose as to permit the arms and legs to be freely stretched, and moved in every direction. It should be succeeded by a loose flannel gown with sleeves, which should be worn till the end of the second month; after which it may be changed to the common clothing used by children of this age."

The advantages of such a dress are, that the movements of the infant will be, as we have already seen, free and unrestrained, and we shall escape the misery of hearing the screams which now so frequently accompany the dressing and undressing of almost every child. No chafings from friction, moreover, can occur; and as the insensible perspiration is in this way promoted over the whole surface of the body, the sympathy between the stomach and skin is happily maintained. A healthy sympathy of this kind, duly kept up, does much towards preserving the stomach in a good state, and the skin from eruptions and sores.

But as I apprehend that christianity is not yet very deeply rooted in the minds and hearts of parents, I have already expressed my doubts whether they are prepared to receive and profit by advice at once rational and physiological. Still I cannot help hoping that I shall succeed in persuading mothers to have every part of a child's dress perfectly loose, except the band already referred to; and that should be but moderately tight.

Common humanity ought to teach us better than to put the body of a helpless infant into a *vise*, and press it to death, as the first mark of our attention. Who has not been struck with a strange inconsistency in the conduct of mothers and nurses, who, while they are so exceedingly tender towards the infant in some points as to injure it by their kindness, are yet almost insensible to its cries of distress while dressing it? So far, indeed, are they from feeling emotions of pity, that they often make light of its cries, regarding them as signs of health and vigor.

There can be no doubt, I confess, that the first cries of an infant, if strong, both indicate and promote a healthy state of the lungs, to a certain extent; but there will always be unavoidable occasions enough for crying to promote health, even after we have done all we can in the way of avoiding pain. They who only draw the child's dress the tighter, the more it cries, are guilty of a crime of little less enormity than murder.

"Think," says Dr. Buchan, "of the immense number of children that die of convulsions soon after birth; and be assured that these (its cries) are much oftener owing to galling pressure, or some external injury, than to any inward cause." This same writer adds, that he has known a child which was "seized with convulsion fits" soon after being "swaddled," immediately relieved by taking off the rollers and bandages; and he says that a loose dress prevented the return of the disease.

I think it is obvious that the utmost extent to which we ought to go, in yielding to the fashion, as it regards form, is to use three pieces of clothing —the shirt, the petticoat and the frock; all of which must be as loose as possible; and before the infant begins to crawl about much, the latter should be long, for the salve of covering the feet and legs. At four or five years of age, loose trowsers, with boys, may be substituted for the petticoat; but it is a question whether something like the frock might not, with every individual, be usefully retained through life.

I wish it were unnecessary, in a book like this, to join in the general complaint against tight lacing any part of the body, but especially the chest. But as this work of torture is sometimes begun almost from the cradle, and as prevention is better than cure, the hope of preventing that for which no cure appears yet to have been found, leads me to make a few remarks on the subject.

As it has long been my opinion that one reason why mothers continue to overlook the subject is, that they do not understand the structure and motion of the chest, I have attempted the following explanation and illustration.

I have already said, that if we bandage tightly, for a considerable time, any part of the human frame, it is apt to become weaker. The more a portion of the frame which is furnished with muscles, those curious instruments of motion, is used, provided it is not *over*-exerted, the more vigorous it is. Bind up an arm, or a hand, or a foot, and keep it bound for twelve hours of the day for many years, and think you it will be as strong as it otherwise would have been? Facts prove the contrary. The Chinese swathe the feet of their infant females; and they are not only small, but weak.

I have said their feet are smaller for being bandaged. So is a hand or an arm. Action—healthy, constant action—is indispensable to the perfect development of the body and limbs. Why it is so, is another thing. But so it is; and it is a principle or law of the great Creator which cannot be evaded. More than this; if you bind some parts of the body tightly, so as to compress them as much as you can without producing actual pain, you will find that the part not only ceases to grow, but actually dwindles away. I have seen this tried again and again. Even the solid parts perish under pressure. When a person first wears a false head of hair, the clasp which rests upon the head, at the upper part of the forehead, being new and elastic, and pressing rather closely, will, in a few months, often make quite an indentation in the cranium or bone of the head.

Now is it probable—nay, is it possible—that the lungs, especially those of young persons, can expand and come to their full and natural size under pressure, even though the pressure should be slight? Must they not be weakened? And if the pressure be strong, as it sometimes is, must they not dwindle away?

We know, too, from the nature and structure of the lungs themselves, that tight lacing must injure them. Many mothers have very imperfect notions of what physicians mean, when they say that corsets impede the circulation, by preventing the full and undisturbed action of the lungs. They get no higher ideas of the *motion* of the *chest,* than what is connected with bending the body forward and backward, from right to left, &c. They know that, if dressed too tightly, *this* motion is not so free as it otherwise would be; but if they are not so closely laced as to prevent that free bending of the body of which I have been speaking, they think there can be no danger; or at least, none of consequence.

Now it happens that this sort of motion is not that to which physicians refer, when they complain of corsets. Strictly speaking, this bending of the whole body is performed by the muscles of the back, and not those of the chest. The latter have very little to do with it. It is true, that even *this* motion ought not to be hindered; but if it is, the evil is one of little comparative magnitude.

Every time we breathe naturally, all the ribs, together with the breast bone, have motion. The ribs rise, and spread a little outward, especially towards the fore part. The breast bone not only rises, but swings forward a little, like a pendulum. But the moment the chest is swathed or bandaged, this motion must be hindered; and the more, in proportion to the tightness.

On this point, those persons make a sad mistake, who say that "a busk not too wide nor too rigid seems to correspond to the supporting spine, and to assist, rather than impede the efforts of nature, to keep the body erect."

Can we seriously compare the offices of the spine with those of the ribs, and suppose that because the former is fixed like a post, at the back part of the lungs, therefore an artificial post in front would be useful? Why, we might just as well argue in favor of hanging weights to a door, or a clog to a pendulum, in order to make it swing backwards and forwards more easily. We might almost as well say that the elbow ought to be made firm, to correspond with the shoulders, and thus become advocates for letting the stays or bandages enclose the arm above the elbow, and fasten it firmly to the side. Indeed, the consequences in the latter case, aside from a little inconvenience, would not be half so destructive to health as in the former.

The ribs, where they join to the back bone, form hinges; and hinges are made for motion. But if you fasten them to a post in front, of what value are the hinges?

If mothers ask, of what use this motion of the lungs is, it is only necessary to refer them to the chapter on Ventilation, in which I trust the subject is made intelligible, and a satisfactory answer afforded.

But I might appeal to facts. Let us look at females around us generally. Do their countenances indicate that they enjoy as good health as they did when dress was worn more loosely? Have they not oftener a leaden hue, as if the blood in them was darker? Are they not oftener short-breathed than formerly? As they advance in life, have they not more chronic diseases? Are not their chests smaller and weaker? And as the doctrine that if one member suffers, all the other members suffer with it, is not less true in physiology than in morals, do we not find other organs besides the lungs weakened? Surgeons and physicians, who, like faithful sentinels, have watched at their post half a century, tell us, moreover, that if these foolish and injurious practices to which I refer are tolerated two centuries longer, every female will be deformed, and the whole race greatly degenerated, physically and morally.

Those with whom no arguments will avail, are recommended to read the following remarks from the first volume of the Library of Health, p. 119:

"It is related, on the authority of Macgill, that in Tunis, after a girl is engaged, or betrothed, she is then *fattened*. For this purpose, she is cooped up in a small room, and shackles of gold and silver are placed upon her ancles and wrists, as a piece of dress. If she is to be married to a man who has discharged, despatched, or lost a former wife, the shackles which the former wife wore are put on the new bride's limbs, and she is fed till they are filled up to a proper thickness. The food used for this custom worthy of the barbarians is called *drough*, which is of an extraordinary fattening quality, and also famous for rendering the milk of the nurse rich and abundant. With this and their national dish, *cuscasoo*, the bride is literally crammed, and many actually die under the spoon."

We laugh at all this, and well we may; but there are customs not very far from home, no less ridiculous.

"There is a country four or five thousand miles westward of Tunis, where the females, to a very great extent, are emaciated for marriage, instead being fattened. This process is begun, in part, by shackles—not of gold and silver, perhaps, but of wood—but instead of being put on loosely, and causing the body or limbs to fill them, they are made to compress the body in the outset; and as the size of the latter diminishes, the shackles are contracted or tightened. As with the eastern, so with the western females, many of them die under the process; though a far greater number die at a remote period, as the consequence of it."

### SEC. 3. *Material.*

I have already committed myself to the reader as favoring the use of soft flannel in cold weather, especially for children who are not yet able to run about freely in the open air. The advantages of an early use of this material, at least for under-clothes, are numerous. The following are a few of them.

1. Flannel, next to the skin, is a pleasant flesh brush; keeping up a gentle and equable irritation, and promoting perspiration and every other function which it is the office of the skin to perform, or assist in performing.

2. It guards the body against the cooling effects of evaporation, when in a state of profuse perspiration.

3. By preventing the heat of the body from escaping too rapidly, it keeps up a steadier temperature on the surface than any other known substance. The importance of the last consideration is greater, in a climate like our own, than elsewhere.

But there are limits to the use of this article of clothing. Whenever the temperature of the atmosphere is so great, even without artificial heat, that we no longer wish to retain the heat of the body by the clothing, then all flannel should be removed at once, and linen should be substituted; taking care to replace the flannel whenever the temperature of the atmosphere, as indicated by the thermometer, or by the child's feelings, may seem to require it.

It should also be kept clean. There is a very general mistake abroad on this subject. Many suppose that flannel can be worn longer without washing than other kinds of cloth. On the contrary, it should be changed oftener than cotton, or even linen, because it will absorb a great deal of fluid, especially the matter of perspiration, which, if long retained, is believed to ferment, and produce unhealthy, if not poisonous gases. For this reason, too, flannel for children's clothing should be white, that it may show dirt the more readily, and obtain the more frequent washing; although it is for this very reason—its liability to exhibit the least particles of dirt—that it is commonly rejected.

One caution more in regard to the use of flannel may be necessary. With some children, owing to a peculiarity of constitution, flannel will produce eruptions on the skin, which are very troublesome. Whenever this is the case, the flannel should be immediately laid aside; upon which the eruptions usually disappear.

If parents would take proper pains to get the lighter, softer kinds of flannel for this purpose, and be particular about its looseness and quantity, I should prefer, as I have already intimated, to have very young children, in our climate, wear this material the greater part of the year, excepting perhaps July and August.

My reasons for this course would be, first, that I like the stimulus of soft flannel on the skin, if changed sufficiently often, better than that of any other kind of clothing. Secondly, cotton is so liable to take fire, that its use in the nursery and among little children seems very hazardous. Thirdly, silk is not quite the appropriate material, as a general thing, besides being too expensive; and fourthly, linen is not warm enough, except in mid-summer.

Except, therefore, in July and August, and in cases of idiosyncracy, such as have just been alluded to, I would use flannel for the under-clothes of young children, throughout the year. But whenever they acquire sufficient strength to walk and run, and play much in the open air, I would gradually lay aside the use of all flannel, even in winter. Great attention, however, must be paid to the *quantity*. The parent who, guided by this rule, should keep on her child the same amount of flannel, and of the same thickness, from January to June 30th, and then, on the first of July, should suddenly exchange it for thin linen, in moderate quantity, might find trouble from it. It is better to make the changes more gradually; otherwise, whatever may be the material of the dress, the child will be likely to suffer.

### SEC. 4. *Quantity.*

The quantity of clothing used by different individuals of the same age, in the same climate, possessing constitutions nearly alike, and following similar occupations, is so different as to strike us with surprise when we first observe the fact.

One will wear nothing but a coarse linen or cotton shirt, coarse coat, waistcoat, and pantaloons, and boots, in the coldest weather. He never, unless it be on the Sabbath, puts on even a cravat, and never in any case stockings or mittens.

Another, in similar circumstances in all respects, constantly wears his thick stockings, flannel wrapper and drawers, and cravat; and seldom goes out, in cold weather, without mittens and an overcoat. He is not a whit warmer: indeed he often suffers more from the cold, than his neighbor who dresses in the manner just described.

Why all this difference? It is no doubt the result of habit. Any individual may accustom himself to much or little clothing. And the earlier the habit is begun, the greater is its influence.

Some persons, observing how little clothing one may accustom himself to use and yet be comfortable, have told us, that so far as mere temperature is concerned, we need no clothing at all. They relate the story of the Scythian and Alexander. Alexander asked the former how he could go without clothes in such a cold climate. He replied, by asking Alexander how he could go with his face naked. "Habit reconciles us to this;" was the reply. "Think me, then, *all* face," said the Scythian.

But admitting that certain individuals, and even a few rude tribes, have gone without clothing; did they therefore follow, in this respect, the intentions of nature? The greatest stickler for adhering to nature's plan, cannot prove this. Analogy is against it. Most of the other animals, even in hot climates, are furnished with a hairy covering from the first; and in cold climates, the Author of their being has even provided them with an increase of clothing for the winter. Their fur, on the approach of cold weather, not only becomes whiter, and therefore conducts the heat away from the body more slowly, but, as every dealer in furs well understands, it becomes softer and thicker. And yet the blood of the furred animals of cold countries is as warm as ours, if not warmer.

The inferences which it seems to me we ought to make from this are, that if other animals require clothing, and even a change of clothing, so does man; and that as the Creator has left him to provide, by his own ingenuity, for a great many of his wants, instead of furnishing him with instinct to direct him, so in relation to dress. And even if it could be proved that dress were naturally unnecessary, with reference to temperature, I should still defend its use on other principles. The few speculative minds, therefore, that in the vagaries of their fancy, but never in their practice, reject it, are not to be regarded.

The principle laid down in the commencement of the chapter on Temperature, is the great principle which should guide us in regard to dress. But although we should always keep a little too cool rather than a little too warm, it is by no means desirable to be cold. Any degree of chilliness, long continued, interrupts the functions which the skin ought to perform, and thus produces mischief.

The same rules, in this respect, apply to eating, as well as to dress. It is better to eat a little less than nature requires, than a little more. It is a generally received opinion, however, that mankind frequently, at least in this country, eat about twice as much as health requires. This is owing to habit; and perhaps the power of the latter is as great in this respect as in regard to dress.

The great point in regard to food or dress is, to *begin* right, and, observing what nature requires—studying at the same time the testimony of others—to endeavor to keep within the bounds she has assigned. It has already been more than intimated, that if the nursery be kept in a proper temperature, a single loose piece of dress is, for some time, all that is required. In pursuance of this principle, through life, I believe few persons would be found who would need more at one time than a single suit of woollen clothes, even in the severest winters of our northern climate.

I have always observed that they who wear the greatest amount of clothing, are most subject to colds. There are obvious reasons why it should be so. This, then, if a fact, is one of the strongest reasons in favor of acquiring a habit of going as thinly clad as we possibly can, and not at the same time feel any inconvenience.

But after all, whether it be winter or summer, we must vary our clothing with the variations of the weather, as indicated by the thermometer, and our own feelings. Sometimes, in our ever-changing and ever-changeable climate, it may be necessary to vary our dress three or four times a day. Some cry out against this practice as dangerous, but I have never found it so. I have known persons who made it a constant practice; and I never found that they sustained any injury from it, except the loss of a little time; and the increase of comfort was more than enough to compensate for that. There is one thing to be avoided, however, whether we change our clothing —our linen especially—twice a day, or only twice a week—which is, *dampness.*

## SEC. 5. *Caps.*

The practice of putting caps on infants is happily going by; and perhaps it may be thought unnecessary for me to dwell a single moment on the subject. But as the practice still prevails in some parts of the country, it may be well to bestow upon it a few passing remarks.

Many mothers have not considered that the circulation of the blood in young infants is peculiarly active; that a large amount of blood is at that period carried to the head; that in consequence of this, the head is proportionably hotter than in adults; and that from this source arises the tendency of very young children to brain-fever, dropsy in the head, and other diseases of this part of the system. But these are most undoubted facts.

Hence one reason why the heads of infants should be kept as cool as possible; and though a thin cap confines less heat than a thick head of hair does when they are older, yet they are less able to bear it. The truth is, that nature furnishes a covering for the head, just about as fast as a covering is required, and the child's safety will permit.

At the present day, few persons will probably be found, who will defend the utility of caps, any longer than till the hair is grown. The general apology for their use after this period, and indeed in most instances before, is, that they look pretty. "What would people say to see my darling without a cap?"

But when the head is kept, from the first, totally uncovered, the hair grows more rapidly, dandruff and other scurfy diseases rarely attack the scalp; catarrh, snuffles, and other similar complaints, and above all, dropsy in the head, seldom show themselves; and the period of cutting teeth, that most dangerous period in the life of an infant, is passed over with much more safety.

"Nothing but custom," says a foreign writer, "can reconcile us to the cap, with all its lace and trumpery ornaments, on the beautiful head of a child; and I would ask any one to say candidly, whether he thinks the children in the pictures of Titian and Raffaelle would be improved by having their heads covered with caps, instead of the silken curls—the adornment of nature—which cluster round their smiling faces. If there were no other reason for disusing caps for infants, but the improvement which it produces in the *appearance* of the child, I would maintain that this is a sufficient inducement." And I concur with him fully.

As to the notion—now I hope nearly exploded—that it is necessary to cover up the "open of the head," as it is called, nothing can be more idle. This part of the head requires no more covering than any other part; and if it did, all the dress in the world could not affect it in the least, except to retard the growth of the bones, which, in due time, ought to close up the space; and this effect, anything which keeps the head too hot might help to produce. Of the folly of wetting the head with spirits, or any other medicated lotions, and of making daily efforts to bring it into shape, it is unnecessary to speak in the present chapter.

## SEC. 6. *Hats and Bonnets.*

The hats worn in this country are almost universally too warm. But if it is a great mistake in adults to wear thick, heavy hats, it is much more so in the case of children.

The infant in the nursery, as we have already seen, needs no covering of the kind. It is absolutely necessary that the head should be kept as cool as possible; and absolutely dangerous to cover it too warmly. At a later period, however, the danger greatly diminishes, because the circulation of the blood becomes more equal, and does not tend so much towards the brain.

Still, however, the head is hotter than the limbs, especially the hands and feet; and I cannot help thinking that the hair is the only covering which is perfectly safe, either in childhood or age; except in the sunshine or in the storm. There may be—there probably is—some danger in going without hat or bonnet in the hot sun; though I have known many children, and some grown persons, who were constantly exposed in this way, and yet appeared not to suffer from it.

But this may be the proper place to state that we are ever in great danger of deceiving ourselves on this subject. If the individuals who follow practices usually regarded as pernicious, while their habits in other respects are just like those of other persons around them who have similar strength, &c. of constitution,—if these individuals, I say, were wholly to escape disease, through life, or if they were to be so much more free from it, and live to an age so much greater than others as to constitute a striking and obvious difference in their favor, we might then safely argue that the practices which they follow are at least without dangers, if not of obvious advantage. But when we see them beset with ills, like other people, it is not safe to pronounce their habits favorable to health, since it is impossible to know whether some of the ills which they suffer are not produced by them.

These remarks are applicable to the disuse of any covering for the head in the sun and in the rain. For you will find those who adopt this practice from early infancy,[Footnote: I say, from early infancy; because we may adopt the best habits in mature years, after our constitutions have been broken up by error and vice, without effecting anything more than to keep us from actually sinking at once. Indeed, in most cases we ought not to expect more.] subject to as many diseases as those around them with similar constitutions, but with habits somewhat different; and as our diseases are generally the consequences of our errors in one way or another, it is impossible to say with certainty that some of them might not have arisen from exposure of the head.

I should not hesitate, therefore, to advise all mothers to put a light hat or bonnet on the heads of their children, whenever they are to be exposed to the direct rays of the summer sun, or to the rain. And as we cannot always foresee when and where these exposures will arise, and as it is believed that these coverings, if light, will never be productive of much injury while we are abroad in the open air, it will follow that it is better to wear than to omit them.

But while I contend for their use as consistent with health and sound philosophy, I must not be understood as admitting the use of such hats as are worn at present, even by children. They are, as I have said before, too hot. What should be substituted, I am unable to determine; but until something can be supplied, which would not be half so oppressive as our common wool hats, I should regard it as the lesser evil to omit them entirely. The danger of going bare-headed, if the practice is commenced early, we know from the customs of some savage nations, can never be very great.

## SEC. 7. *Covering for the Feet.*

The same reason for avoiding the use of any covering for the head, in early infancy, is a sufficient reason for covering the feet well. For just in proportion as the blood is sent to the head in superabundance, and keeps up in it an undue degree of heat, just in the same proportion is it sent to the feet in too *small* a quantity, leaving these parts liable to cold. Now it is a fundamental law with medical men, that the feet ought to be kept warmer than the head, if possible; especially while the child is very young, and exposed to brain diseases.

So long, therefore, as children are young, and unable to exercise their feet, stockings ought to be used, both in summer and winter; but I prefer to have them short, unless long ones can be used without garters. Everything in the shape of a garter or ligature round the limbs, body, or neck of a child, except a single body-band, already mentioned in another chapter, ought forever to be banished.

It has often been objected, I know, that stockings will make the feet tender. But as no child was ever hardened by *continued* and severe cold applied to any part of the body, but the contrary, so no one was ever made more tender by being kept moderately warm. Excess of heat, like excess of cold, will alike weaken either children or adults; but there is little danger of heating the feet and legs of infants too much during the first year of infancy.

It is also said that stockings are apt to receive and retain wet. But as I shall show in another place that wet clothes should be frequently changed, this objection would be equally strong against wearing coats and diapers.

As to shoes, there is some variety of opinion among medical men. A few hold that they cramp the feet, and prevent children from learning to walk as early as they otherwise would. If it were best for children that they should learn to walk as early as possible, the last objection might have weight. But it seems to me not at all desirable to be in haste about their walking. Indeed, I greatly prefer to retard their progress, in this respect, rather than to hasten it.

As to the first objection, that shoes cramp the feet too much, nearly its whole force turns upon the question whether they are made of proper materials or not. There is no need of making them of cow-hide, or any other thick leather. The soles are the most important part. These will defend the feet against pins, needles, and such other sharp substances as are usually found on the floor; and the upper part of the shoe, so long as the wearer remains in the nursery, may be made of the softest and most yielding material—even of cloth. Infants' shoes should always be made on two lasts, one for each foot.

The philosopher Locke held, that in order to harden the young, their shoes ought to be "so that they might leak and let in water, whenever they came near it." There may be and probably is, no harm in having a child wet his feet occasionally, provided he is soon supplied with dry stockings again; but it is hazardous for either children or adults to go too long in wet stockings, and especially to sit long in them, after they have been using much active exercise. I am in favor of good, substantial shoes and stockings for people of all ages and conditions, and at all seasons; and believe it entirely in accordance with sound economy and the laws of the human constitution.

## SEC. 8. *Pins.*

The custom of using ten or a dozen pins in the dressing of children, ought by all means to be set aside. They not only often wound the skin, but they have occasionally been known to penetrate the body and the joints of the limbs. So many of these dreadful accidents occur, and where no accident happens, so much pain is occasionally given by their sharp points to the little sufferer, who cannot tell what the matter is, that it is quite time the practice were abolished.

Do you ask what can be substituted?—The following mode is adopted by Dr. Dewees in his own family, as mentioned in his work on the "Physical and Medical Treatment of Children," at page 86.

"The belly-band and the petticoat have strings; and not a single pin is used in their adjustment. The little shirt, which is always made much larger than the infant's body, is folded on the back and bosom, and these folds kept in their places by properly adjusting the body of the petticoat: so far not a pin is used. The diaper requires one, but this should be of a large size, and made to serve the double purpose of holding the folds of this article, as well as keeping the belly-band in its proper place; the latter having a small tag of double linen depending from its lower margin, by which it is secured to the diaper, by the same pin.

"Should an extraordinary display of best 'bib and tucker' be required upon any special occasion, a third pin may be admitted to ensure the well-sitting of the 'frock' waist in front;—this last pin, however, is applied externally; so that the risk of its getting into the child's body is very small, even if it should become displaced."

The writer from whom the last two paragraphs are taken, says be has seen needles substituted for pins; and relates a long story of a child whose life was well nigh destroyed in this manner. It underwent months of ill health, and many moments of excruciating agony, before the cause of its trouble was suspected. Sometimes its distress was so great that nothing but large doses of laudanum, sufficient to stupify it, could afford the least relief. At last a tumor was discovered by the attending physician, near one of the bones on which we sit, and a needle was extracted two inches long. The needle had been put in its clothes, and, by slipping into the folds of the skin, had insinuated itself, unperceived, into the child's body. It is pleasing to add, that, although the little sufferer had now been ill seven or eight months, and had endured almost everything but death,—fever, diarrhoea, and the most excruciating pain,—it soon recovered.

This shocking circumstance is enough, one would think, to deter every mother or nurse, who becomes acquainted with it, from using needles in infants' clothes. Happy would it be, if, in banishing needles, they would contrive to banish pins also, and adopt either the plan of Dr. Dewees, or one still more rational.

### SEC. 9. *Remaining Wet.*

On the subject of changing the wet clothing of a child, there is a strange and monstrous error abroad; which is, that by suffering them to remain wet and cold, we harden the constitution. The filthiness of this practice is enough to condemn it, were there nothing else to be said against it.

It is insisted on by many, I know, that as water which is salt, when it is applied to the skin, and suffered to remain long, while it secures the point of hardening the child, prevents all possibility of its taking cold, it hence follows, that wet diapers are not injurious. But this is a mistake. Every time an infant is allowed to remain wet, we not only endanger its taking cold, but expose it to excoriations of the skin, if not to serious and dangerous inflammation. In short, if frequent changes are not made, whatever some mothers and nurses may think, they may rest assured, that the health of the child must sooner or later suffer as the consequence.

Nor is it enough to hang up a diaper by the fire, and, as soon as it is dry, apply it again. It should be clean, as well as dry. Let us not be told, that it is troublesome to wash so often. Everything is in a certain sense troublesome. Everything in this world, which is worth having, is the result of toil. Nothing but absolute poverty affords the shadow of an excuse for neglecting anything which will promote the health, or even the comfort of the tender infant.

Of the impropriety and danger of suffering wet clothes to dry upon us, I shall speak elsewhere; as well as of the evil of suffering children to remain dirty,—their skins or their clothing.

### SEC. 10. *Remarks on the Dress of Boys.*

Whatever tends to disturb the growth of the body, or hinder the free exercise of the limbs, during the infancy and childhood of both sexes is injurious. And as every mother has the control of these things, I have thought it desirable to append to this chapter a few thoughts on the particular dress of each sex. I begin with that of boys.

"Nothing can be more injurious to health," says a foreign writer, "than the tight jacket, buttoned up to the throat, the well-fitted boots, and the stiff stock." And his remarks are nearly as applicable to this country as to England. The consequences of this preposterous method of dressing boys, are diminutive manhood, deformity of person, and a constitution either already imbued with disease, or highly susceptible of its impression.

No part of the modern dress of boys is more absurd, than the stiff stock, or thick cravat. It is not only injurious by pressing on the *jugular* veins, and preventing the blood from freely passing out of the head, but, by constantly pressing on the numerous and complex muscles of the neck, at this period of life, it prevents their development; because whatever hinders the action of the muscular parts, hinders their growth, and makes them even appear as if wasted.

It would be a great improvement, if this part of dress were wholly discarded; and when is there so appropriate a time for setting it aside, as *before we began to use it*; or rather while we are under the more immediate care of our mothers?

The use of jackets buttoned up to the throat, except in cold weather, is objectionable; but this is very fortunately going out of fashion.

Boots, if used at all, should fit well; to this there can be no possible objection. What the writer, whom I have quoted, referred to, was probably the tight boot, worn to prevent the foot from being large and unseemly; but producing, as tight boots inevitably do, an injurious effect upon the muscles, a constrained walk, and corns.

What can be more painful, than to see little boys—yes, *little* boys—boys neither fifteen, nor twenty, nor twenty-five, walk as if they were fettered and trussed up for the spit; unable to look down, or turn their heads, on account of a thick stock, or two or three cravats piled on the top of each other—and only capable of using their arms to dangle a cane, or carry an umbrella, as they hobble along, perhaps on a hot sun-shiny day in July or August?

But this evil, you who are mothers, have it very generally in your power to prevent, if you are only wise enough to secure that ascendancy over your children's minds which the Author of their nature designed. At the least, you can prevent it for a time—the most important period, too—by your own authority. This you will not need any urging to induce you to do, if you ever become thoroughly convinced of its pre-eminent folly.

### SEC. 11. *On the Dress of Girls.*

The same general principles which should guide the young mother in regard to the dress of boys, are equally important and applicable in the management of girls. The whole dress should, as much as possible, hang loosely from the shoulders, without pressing on the body, or any part of it. This, I say, is the grand point to be aimed at; and this is the only great principle, whatever some mothers may think, which will lead to true beauty of person, and gracefulness of gesture.

There is, however, a slight difference to be made between the dress of girls and that of boys. The greater delicacy of the female frame requires that the surface of the body should be kept rather warmer, as well as better protected from the vicissitudes of the atmosphere.

But is this the fact? Is not the contrary true? While boys in the winter are clad in warm woollen vestments, covering every part of their trunk, many portions of the female frame, and especially many parts of their limbs, are left so much exposed, that in cold weather you scarcely find a girl abroad, who appears to be comfortable.

Nay, they are not only uncomfortable abroad, but at home; and if I were to present to mothers in detail, a tenth of the evils which their daughters suffer from not adopting a warmer method of clothing, I should probably be stared at by some, and laughed at by others. All this, too, without speaking of going out of warm concert rooms, theatres, ball rooms and lecture rooms, into the night air, or out of school rooms and churches, to walk home with measured and stiffened pace, lest the sin unpardonable of walking swiftly or RUNNING,—that active exercise which health requires, which youthful feeling prompts, and which duty ought to inspire,—should unwarily be committed.

The tremendous evils of confining the lungs have been adverted to at sufficient length. In reference to that general subject, I need only add, that if the chest be not duly exercised and expanded, the liver, the lungs, the stomach, digestion, absorption, circulation and perspiration, are all hindered. And even so far as the various internal organs of the body *are* active, they act at a great disadvantage. The blood which they "work up," is bad blood, and must be so, as long as the lungs do not have free play. Hence may and do arise all sorts of diseases; especially diseases of OBSTRUCTION; and such as are often very difficult of removal.

What can be a more pitiable sight than some modern girls going home from school or church in winter? Thinly clad, the blood is all driven from the surface upon the internal organs, and what remains is so loaded with carbon, which the lungs ought but cannot discharge, that her skin has a leaden hue; her teeth chatter; her very heart is chilled in her panting, frozen bosom; she cannot run, and if she could, she must not, for it would be vulgar! Every mother should shrink from the sight of such a picture.

---

# CHAPTER V.

## CLEANLINESS.

*Physiology of the human skin. Of checking perspiration. Diseases thus produced. "Dirt" not "healthy." How the mistake originated. "Smell of the earth." Effect of uncleanliness on the morals. Filthiness produces bowel complaints. Changing dress for the sake of cleanliness.*

No mother will ever pay that attention to cleanliness which its importance to health and happiness demands, till she perceives its necessity. And she will never perceive that necessity till she has studied attentively the machinery of the human frame—and especially its wonderful covering.

The skin is pierced with little openings or *pores*, so numerous that some have reckoned them at a million to every square inch. At all events, they are so small that the naked eye can neither distinguish nor count them; and so numerous, that we cannot pierce the skin with the finest needle without hitting one or more of them.

When we are in perfect health, and the skin clean, a gentle moisture or mist continually oozes through these pores. This process is called *perspiration*; and the moisture which thus escapes, the *matter* of perspiration.

Perspiration may be checked in two ways. 1. by filth on the skin; 2. by what is commonly called taking cold—for taking cold essentially consists in chilling the skin to such a degree as to stop, for some time, the escape of this moisture. Most persons have doubtless observed, that in the first stages of a cold, they frequently have a very dry skin. Whereas, when we are in health, the skin usually feels moist.

Our health is not only endangered, and a foundation laid for fevers, rheumatisms, and consumptions, by stopping the pores of the skin with dirt, or anything else, but there is also danger from another and a very different source.

The blood, in its circulation through the body, is constantly becoming impure; and as it thus comes back impure to the heart, is as constantly sent to the lungs, where it comes in close contact with the air which we breathe, and is purified. But this same purifying process which goes on in the lungs, goes on, too, if the skin is in a pure, free, healthy condition, all over the surface of the body. If it is not—if the skin cannot do this part of the work—an additional burden is thus laid on the lungs, which in this way soon become so overworked, that they cannot perform their own proportion of the labor. And whenever this happens, the health must soon suffer.

The strange belief, that "dirt is healthy," has much influence on the daily practice of thousands of those who are ignorant of the human structure, and the laws which govern and regulate the animal economy. It has probably originated in the well-known fact, that those children who are allowed to play in the dirt, are often as healthy—and even *more* healthy—than those who are confined to the nursery or the parlor.

Now, while it is admitted that this is a very common case, it is yet believed that the former class of children would be still more vigorous than they now are, if they were kept more cleanly, or were at least frequently washed. It is not the dirt which promotes their health, but their active exercise in the open air; the advantages of which are more than sufficient to compensate for the injury which they sustain from the dirt. That is to say, they retain, in spite of the dirt, better health than those who are denied the blessings of pure air and abundant exercise, and subjected to the opposite extreme of almost constant confinement.

There is something deceitful, after all, in the ruddy, blooming appearance of those children who are left by the busy parent to play in the road or field, without attention to cleanliness. If this were not so, how comes it to pass that they suffer much more, not only from chronic, but from acute diseases, than children whose parents are in better circumstances?

I am the more solicitous to combat a belief in the salutary tendency of an unclean skin, because I know it prevails to some extent; and because I know also, both from reason and from fact, that it is a gross error.

It is, however, true, that years sometimes intervene, before the evil consequences of dirtiness appear. The office of the vessels of the skin being interrupted, an increase of action is imposed on other parts, especially on those internal organs commonly called glands, which action is apt to settle into obstinate disease. Hence, at least when aided by other causes, often arise, in later life, after the source of the evil is forgotten, if it were ever suspected, rheumatism, scrofula, jaundice, and even consumption.

There is a strange notion abroad, that the *smell* of the earth is beneficial, especially to consumptive persons. I honestly believe, however, that it is more likely to create consumption than to cure it. Besides, in what does this smell consist? Do the silex, the alumine, and the other earths, with their compounds, emit any odor? Rarely, I believe, unless when mixed with vegetable matter. But no gases necessary to health are evolved during the decomposition of vegetable matter; on the contrary, it is well known that many of them tend to induce disease.

I am thoroughly persuaded that too much attention cannot be paid to cleanliness; and the demand for such attention is equally imperious in the case of those who cultivate the earth, or labor in it, or on stone, during the intervals of their useful avocations, as in the case of those individuals who follow other employments.

I must also protest against the doctrine, that the smell or taste of the earth, much less a coat of it spread over the surface, and closing up, for hours and days together, thousands and millions of those little pores with which the Author of this "wondrous frame" has pierced the skin, can have a salutary tendency.

The opinion has been even maintained, that uncleanly habits are not only unfavorable to health, but to morality. There can be no doubt that he who neglects his person and dress will be found lower in the scale of morals, other things being equal, than he who pays a due regard to cleanliness.

Some have supposed that a disposition to neglect personal cleanliness was indicative of genius. But this opinion is grossly erroneous, and has well nigh ruined many a young man.

I am far from recommending any degree of fastidiousness on this subject. Truth and correct practice usually lie between extremes. But I do and must insist, that the connection between cleanliness of body and purity of moral character, is much more close and direct than has usually been supposed.

But to return to the more immediate effects of cleanliness on health. There is one class of diseases in particular which, in an eminent degree, owe their origin to a neglect of cleanliness. I refer to the bowel complaints so common among children during summer and autumn. Except in case of teething, the use of unripe fruits, or the *abuse* of those which are in themselves excellent, it is probable that more than half of the bowel complaints of the young are either produced or greatly aggravated by a foul skin.

The importance of washing the whole body in water will be insisted on in the chapter on Bathing; it is therefore unnecessary to say anything farther on that subject in this place, except to observe that whether the washings of the body be partial or general, they should be thorough, so far as they are carried. There are thousands of children who, in pretending to wash their hands and face, will do little more than wet the inside of their hands, and the tips of their noses and ears unless great care is taken.

Few things are more important than suitable changes of dress. There are those, who, from principle, never wear the same under-garment but one day without washing, either in summer or winter; and there are others who, though they may wear an article without washing two or three successive days, take care to change their dress at night—never sleeping in a garment which they have worn during the day.

It is a very common objection to suggestions like these, that they will do very well for those who have wealth, but not for the poor;—that *they* have neither the time nor the means of attending to them. How can they change their clothes every day? we are asked. And how can they afford to have a separate dress for the night?

# CHAPTER VI.

## ON BATHING.

Danger of savage practices. Rousseau. Cold water at birth. First washing of the child. Rules. Temperature. Bathing vessels. Unreasonable fears. Whims. Views of Dr. Dewees. Hardening. Rules for the cold bath. Securing a glow. Coming out of the bath. Local baths. Shower bath. Vapor bath. Sponging. Neglect of bathing The Romans. Treatment of children compared with that of domestic animals.

Some of the hardy nations of antiquity, as well as a few savage tribes of modern times, have been accustomed to plunge their new-born infants into cold water. This is done for the two-fold purpose of washing and hardening them.

To all who reason but for a moment on this subject, the danger of such a practice must be obvious. So sudden a change from a temperature of nearly 100° of Fahrenheit to one quite low, perhaps scarcely 40°, must and does have a powerful effect on the nervous system even of an adult; but how much more on that of a tender infant? We may form some idea of this, by the suddenness and violence of its cries, by the sudden contractions and relaxations of its limbs and body, and by its palpitating heart and difficult breathing.

Every one's experience may also remind him, that what produces at best a momentary pain to himself, cannot otherwise than be painful to the infant. In making a comparison between adults and infants, however, in this respect, we should remember that the lungs of the infant do not get into full and vigorous action until some time after birth; and that, on this account, the hold they have on life is so feeble, that any powerful shock, and especially that given by the cold bath, is ten times more dangerous to them than to adults, or even to infants themselves, after a few months have elapsed.

It is surprising to me that so sensible a writer as Rousseau generally is on education, should have encouraged this dangerous practice; and still more so that many fathers even now, blinded by theory, should persist in it, notwithstanding the pleadings of the mother or the nurse, and the plainest dictates of common sense and common prudence.[Footnote: Nothing is intended to be said here, which shall encourage unthinking nurses or mothers in setting themselves against measures which have been prescribed by higher authority,—I mean the physician. There are cases of this kind, where it requires all the resolution which a father, uninterrupted, can summon to his aid, to administer a dose or perform a task, on which he knows the existence of his child may be depending: but when the thoughtless entreaties of the mother or nurse are interposed, it makes his condition most distressing. Mothers, in such cases, ought to encourage rather than remonstrate. They who *do not*, are guilty of cruelty, and—perhaps—of infanticide.]

A child plunged into cold water at birth, by those whose theories carry them so far as to do it even in the coldest weather, has sometimes been twenty-four hours in recovering, notwithstanding the most active and judicious efforts to restore it. In other instances the results have been still more distressing. Dr. Dewees is persuaded that he has "known death itself to follow the use of cold water," in this way—I believe he means *immediate* death—and adds, with great confidence, that he has "repeatedly seen it require the lapse of several hours before reaction could establish itself; during which time the pale and sunken cheeks and livid lips declared the almost exhausted state" of the infant's excitability.[Footnote: "Dewees on children" p. 72.]

We need not hesitate to put very great confidence in the opinion here expressed; for besides being a close and just observer of human nature, Dr. D. has had the direction and management, in a greater or less degree, of several thousands of new-born infants.

Nothing, indeed, in the whole range of physical education, seems better proved, than that while some few infants, whose constitutions are naturally very strong, are invigorated by the practice in question, others, in the proportion of hundreds for one, who are *less* robust, are injured for life; some of them seriously.

Nor will spirits added to the water make any material difference. I am aware that there is a very general notion abroad, that the injurious effects of cold water, in its application both internally and externally, are greatly diminished by the addition of a little spirit; but it is not so. Does the addition of such a small quantity of spirit as is generally used in these cases, materially alter the temperature? Is it not the application of a cold liquid to a heated surface, still? Can we make anything else of it, either more or less?

I do not undertake to say, that the cold bath may not be so managed in the progress of infancy, as to make it beneficial, especially to strong constitutions. It is its indiscriminate application to all new-born children, without regard to strength of constitution, or any other circumstances, that I most strenuously oppose. Of its occasional use, under the eye of a physician, and by parents who will discriminate, I shall say more presently.

Our first duty on receiving a new inhabitant of the world is, to see that it is gently but thoroughly washed, in moderately warm soft water, with fine soap. Special attention should be paid to the folds of the joints, the neck, the arm pits, &c. For rubbing the body, in order to disengage anything which might obstruct the pores, or irritate or fret the skin, nothing can be preferable to a piece of soft sponge or flannel. Though the operation should be thorough, and also as rapid as the nature of circumstances will permit, all harshness should be avoided. When finished, the child should be wiped perfectly dry with soft flannel.

While the washing is performed, the temperature of the room should be but a few degrees lower than that of the water; and the child should not be exposed to currents of cold air. If the weather is severe, or if currents of air in the room cannot otherwise be avoided, the dressing, undressing, washing, &c., may be done near the fire. And I repeat the rule, it should always be done with as much rapidity as is compatible with safety.

Here will be seen one great advantage of simplicity in the form of dress. If the more rational suggestions of our chapter on that subject are attended to, it will greatly facilitate the process of washing, and the subsequent daily process of bathing, which I am about to recommend to my readers.

This washing process is also an introduction to bathing. For it should be repeated every day; but with less and less attention to the washing, and more and more reference to the bathing. How long the child should stay in the bath, must be left to experience. If he is quiet, fifteen minutes can never be too long; and I should not object to twenty. If otherwise, and you are obliged to remove him in five minutes, or even in three, still the bathing will be of too much service to be dispensed with.

Nothing should be mixed with the water, if the infant is healthy, except a little soap, as already mentioned. Some are fond of using salt; but it is by no means necessary, and may do harm.

The proper hour for bathing is the early part of the day, or about the middle of the forenoon. This season is selected, because the process, manage it as carefully as we may, is at first a little exhausting. As the child grows older, however, and not only becomes stronger, but appears to be actually refreshed and invigorated by the bath, it will be advisable to defer it to a later and later hour. By the time the babe is three months old, particularly in the warm season, the hour of bathing may be at sunset.

The degree of heat must be determined, in part, by observing its effect on the child; and in part by a thermometer. For this, and for other purposes, a thermometer, as I have already more than hinted, is indispensable in every nursery. Our own sensations are often at best a very unsafe guide. There is one rule which should always be observed—never to have the temperature of the bath below that of the air of the room. If the thermometer show the latter to be 70°, the bath should be something like 80° perhaps with feeble children, rather more.

Great care ought always to be taken to proportion the air of the room and the water of the bath to each other. If, for example, the temperature of the room have been, for some time, unusually warm, that of the water must not be so low as if it had been otherwise. On the contrary, if the room have been, for a considerable time, rather cool, the bath may be made several degrees cooler than in other circumstances. But in no case and in no circumstances must a *warm* bath—intended as such, simply—be so warm or so cold, as to make the child uncomfortable; whether the temperature be 70°, 80°, or 90°.

It is hardly necessary to add, that in bathing a young child, the vessel used for the purpose should be large enough to give free scope to all the motions of its extremities. Most children are delighted to play and scramble about in the water. I know, indeed, that the contrary sometimes happens; but when it does, it is usually—I do not say *always*—because the countenances of those who are around express fear or apprehension; for it is surprising how early these little beings learn to decipher our feelings by our very countenances.

Some of our readers may be surprised at the intimation that there are mothers and nurses who have fears or apprehensions in regard to the effects of the warm bath; but others—and it is for such that I write this paragraph—will fully understand me. I have been often surprised at the fact, but it is undoubted, that there is a strong prejudice against warm bathing, in many parts of the country. In endeavoring to trace the cause, I have usually found that it arose from having seen or heard of some child who died soon after its application. I have had many a parent remonstrate with me on the danger of the warm bath; and this, too, in circumstances when it appeared to me, that the child's existence depended, under God, on that very measure. Perhaps it is useless in such cases, however, to reason with parents on the subject. The medical practitioner must do his duty boldly and fearlessly, and risk the consequences.

But as I am writing, not for persons under immediate excitement, but for those that may be reasoned with, it is proper to say, that in medicine, the warm bath is so often used in extreme cases, and as a last resort, even when death has already grasped, or is about to fix his grasp on the sufferer, that it would be very strange if many persons *did not* die, just after bathing. But that the bathing itself ever produced this result, in one case in a thousand, there is not the slightest reason for believing. [Footnote: Let me not be understood as intimating that, the general neglect of bathing, of which I complain so loudly, is *chiefly* owing to this unreasonable prejudice, though this no doubt has its sway. On the contrary, I believe it is much oftener owing to ignorance, indolence, and parsimony.]

There are many more whims connected with bathing, as with almost everything else, which it were equally desirable to remove. Some nurses and mothers think that if the child's skin is wiped dry after bathing, it will impair, if not destroy, the good effects of the operation. Others still, shocking to relate, will even put it to bed in its wet clothes; this, too, from principle. Not unlike this, is the belief, very common among adults, that if we get our clothes wet—even our stockings—we must, by all means, suffer them to dry on us; a belief which, in its results, has sent thousands to a premature grave—and, what is still worse, made invalids, for life, of a still greater number.

I am aware, that in rejecting the indiscriminate cold bathing of infants, I am treading on ground which is rather unpopular, even with medical men; a large proportion of whom seem to believe that the practice may be useful. But I am not *wholly* alone. Dr. Dewees—of whose large experience I have already spoken—and some others, do not hesitate to avow similar sentiments.

The objections of Dr. Dewees to cold bathing are the following. 1. There often exists a predisposition to disease, which cold bathing is sure to rouse to action. Or if the disease have already begun to affect the system, the bath is sure to aggravate it. 2. Some children have such feeble constitutions that they are sure to be permanently weakened by it, rather than invigorated. 3. To those in whom there is the tendency of a large quantity of blood to the head, lungs, liver, &c., it is injurious. 4. In some, the shock produces a species of syncope, or catalepsy. 5. The *reaction*, as shown by the heat which follows the cold bath, is, in some cases, so great as to produce a degree of fever, and consequent debility. 6. It never answers the purposes of cleanliness—one great object of bathing—so well as the warm bath. 7. It is always unpleasant or painful to the child; especially at first. 8. It sometimes produces severe pain in the bowels.

This is a very formidable list of objections; and certainly deserves consideration. There is one statement made by Dr. D. in the progress of his remarks on this subject, in which I do not concur. He says—"The object of all bathing is to remove impurities arising from dust, perspiration, &c., from the surface; that the skin may not be obstructed in the performance of its proper offices."

But the object of cold bathing, with many, is to *harden*; consequently it is not true that cleanliness is the *only object*. If he means, even, that cleanliness is the only *legitimate* object of all bathing, I shall still be compelled to dissent.

If the cold bath could be used, always, by and with the direction of a skilful physician, I believe its occasional use might be rendered salutary. And although as it is now commonly used, I believe its effects are almost anything but salutary, I do not deny that if its use were cautiously and gradually begun, and judiciously conducted, it might be the means of making children who are already robust, still more hardy and healthy than before, and better able to resist those sudden changes of temperature so common in our climate, and so apt to produce cold, fever, and consumption.

Cold bathing, in the hands of those who are ignorant of the laws of the human frame—and such unfortunately and unaccountably most fathers and mothers are—I cannot help regarding as a highly dangerous weapon; and therefore it is, that in view of the whole subject, I cannot recommend its general and indiscriminate use.

If there are individuals, however, who are determined to employ it, in the case of their more vigorous children, and without the advice or direction of their family physician, I beg them to attend to the following rules or principles, expressed as briefly as possible.

In no ordinary case whatever, is the cold bath useful, unless it is succeeded by that degree of warmth on the surface of the body which is usually called a *glow*. This is a leading and important principle. The contrary, that is, the injurious effects of cold bathing—its *immediate* bad effects, I mean—are shown by the skin remaining pale and shrivelled after coming out of the bath, by its blue appearance, and by its coldness, as well as by a sunken state of the eyes, and much general languor.

To secure this point—I mean the GLOW—it is indispensably important to begin the use of cold water gradually; that is, to use it at first of so high a temperature as to produce only a slight sensation of cold, and to take special care that the skin be immediately wiped very dry, and the temperature of the room be quite as high as usual. Afterward the water may be cooled gradually, from week to week, though never more than a degree or two at once.

It will probably be unsafe to commence this practice of cold bathing—even in the case of the most robust children—until they are at least six months of age.

The appropriate season will be the middle of the forenoon, the hour when the system is usually the most vigorous, and at which we shall be most likely to secure a reaction. At first, twice or three times a week are as often as it will be safe to repeat it. Some writers recommend it twice a day; but once is enough, under any ordinary circumstances.

The method at first is, to give the infant a single plunge. Afterward, when he becomes older, and more inured to it, he may be plunged several times in succession.

On taking him out of the bath, the skin should be wiped perfectly dry, as in the case of the warm bath, and with the same or an increased degree of attention to other circumstances—the temperature of the room, the avoiding currents of air, &c. He should next be put in a soft, warm blanket, and be kept for some time in a state of gentle motion; and after a little time, should be dressed.

I have already mentioned the importance of avoiding the manifestation of fear, when we bathe a child; and the caution is particularly necessary in the administration of the cold bath. Some writers even recommend, that during the whole process of undressing, bathing, exercising, and dressing, singing should be employed. There is philosophy in this advice, and it is easily tried; but I cannot speak of it from experience.

There is one thing which may serve to calm our apprehensions—if we have any—of danger; which is, that though the child's lungs are feeble at first, from their not having been, like the heart, accustomed to previous action, yet when they get fairly into motion and action, and the child is a few months old, they are probably as strong, if not stronger, in proportion, than those of adults.

Bathing in cold water should never be performed immediately after a full meal. Neither is it desirable to go to the contrary extreme, and bathe when the stomach has been long empty; nor when the child's mental or bodily powers are more than usually exhausted by fatigue.

Although I have given these rules for those who are determined to use the cold bath with their children, yet, for fear I shall be misunderstood, I must be suffered to repeat, in this place, that, uninformed as people generally are in regard to physiology, I cannot advise even its moderate use On the contrary, I would gladly dissuade from it, as most likely, in the way it would inevitably be used, to do more harm than good.

There is no sort of objection to what might be called local bathing with cold water. If the child's head is hot at any time, the temples, and indeed the whole upper part of the head, may be very properly wet with moderately cold water—taking care to avoid wetting the clothes. But avoid, by all means, the common but foolish practice of putting spirits in the water.

A tea-spoonful of cold water cannot be too early put into the mouth of the infant. The object is to cleanse or rinse the mouth; and the process may be aided by wiping it out with a piece of soft linen rag. If a part or all of the water should be swallowed, no harm will be done. This practice, commenced almost as soon as children are born, has saved many a sore mouth.

There are other forms of bathing besides those already mentioned; among which are the shower bath, the vapor bath, and the medicated bath. The shower bath—for which purpose the water is commonly used cold—is but poorly adapted to the wants of infants. The shock is much greater than the common cold bath, and more apt to frighten; and fear is unfavorable to reaction, or the production of a genial glow.

The vapor bath is much better; and probably has quite as good an effect as the common warm bath. The trouble and expense of procuring the necessary apparatus is somewhat greater, however, as a mere bathing tub costs but little, and can be made by every father who possesses common ingenuity. But whatever may be the expense, it is indispensable in every family; and whenever the pores of the skin are obstructed, a vapor bathing apparatus is equally desirable.

The medicated vapor bath is sometimes used; but I am not now treating of infants who are sick, but of those who are in a state of health.

The common warm bath is sometimes medicated by putting in salt. This, of course, renders the water more stimulating to the skin; but except when the perspiration is checked, or the skin peculiarly inactive from some other cause—in other words, unless we are sick—it is seldom expedient to use it.

There is one substitute for the bathing tub, in the case of the cold bath. I refer to the use of a wet cloth or sponge, applied rapidly to the whole surface of the body. When this is done, the skin should be wiped thoroughly dry immediately afterwards, as in the case of complete immersion.

The application of either a cloth or a sponge, filled with warm water, to the skin, in this manner, even if continued for several minutes together, is less efficacious than a continuous immersion. I repeat it—no family ought to be without conveniences for bathing in warm water daily. I speak now of every member of the family, young and old, as well as the infant; and I refer particularly to the summer season: though I do not think the practice ought to be wholly discontinued during the winter.

It will still be objected that this care of, and attention to the young, in reference to health—this provision for bathing daily, and care to see that it is performed—can never be afforded by the laboring portion of the community. But I shall as strenuously insist on the contrary; and trust I shall, in the sequel, produce reasons which will be satisfactory.

The great difficulty is, to convince parents that these things are vastly more productive of health and happiness to their children—more truly necessaries—than a great many things for which they now expend their time and money. There is, and always has been—except, perhaps, among the Jews, in the earliest periods of the history of that wonderful nation—a strange disposition to overlook the happiness of the young. It is not necessary to represent this dereliction as peculiar to modern times, for we find traces of the same thing thousands of years ago.

The Roman emperors—Dioclesian in particular—could make provision for bathing, to an extent which now astonishes us; but for whom? For whom, I repeat it, was incurred the enormous expense of fitting up and keeping in repair accommodations for bathing at once 18,000 people? For adults; and for adults alone. I do not say that children were not admitted, in any case; but I say they were not contemplated in these arrangements. Nothing was done—not a single thing—that would not have been done, had there been no child under ten years of age in the whole empire.

And what better than this do WE, now? We make provision for the happiness of the adult. The most indigent person will find time and money to spend for the gratification of his own senses, his pride, or his curiosity; but his children—they may be overlooked! Or, if he has an eye to the future happiness of his child, he conceives that he is promoting it in the best possible degree, by endeavoring to lay up a few dollars for his use, after his character is formed—at a period, as it too often happens, when money will do him little good, since it can neither purchase health, peace of mind, nor reputation.

Far be it from me to say, that the poor—ground into the dust as they are, by the force of circumstances operating with their own concurrence, to make them ignorant, vicious, or miserable—can do for their children all that is desirable. By no means. But they have it in their power to do much more than they are at present doing. They have it in their power, at least, to use the same good sense in the management of the human being that they do in that of a pig, a calf, or a colt, or even a young vegetable. No parent, let him be ever so poor, is found in the habit of neglecting either of these in proportion to its infancy, and of exerting himself only in proportion as it grows older. Common sense tells him that the contrary is the true course; that however poor he may be, he will be still poorer, if he do not take special pains with the young animal, to rear it and with the young vegetable, to give it the right direction, by keeping down the weeds, and pruning and watering it. And I say again, that however deserving of censure the wealthy of a Christian community may be in not directing the ignorant and vicious into the right path, and in not expending more of their wealth on those who are poor, in elevating their minds and their manners, and promoting their health, still the latter are inexcusable for their present neglect of their infant offspring, while they would not think of neglecting, on the same principle, the offspring of their domestic animals.

# CHAPTER VII.

## FOOD.

SEC. 1. General principles.—SEC. 2. Conduct of the mother.—SEC. 3. Nursing—rules in regard to it.—SEC. 4. Quantity of food. Errors. Over-feeding. Gluttony.—SEC. 5. How long should milk be the child's only food?—SEC. 6 Feeding before teething. Cow's milk. Sucking bottles. Cleanliness. Nurses.—SEC. 7. Treatment from teething to weaning.—SEC. 8. Process of weaning-rules in regard to it.—SEC. 9. First food to be used after weaning. Importance of good bread. Other kinds of food.—SEC. 10. Remarks on fruit.—SEC. 11. Evils and dangers of confectionary.—SEC. 12. Mischiefs of pastry.—SEC. 13. Crude and raw substances.

### SEC. 1. *General Principles.*

The mother's milk, in suitable quantity, and under suitable regulations, is so obviously the appropriate food of an infant during the first months of its existence, that it seems almost unnecessary to repeat the fact. And yet the violations of this rule are so numerous and constant, as to require a few passing remarks.

There are some mothers who seem to have a perfect hatred of children; and if they can find any plausible apology for neglecting to nurse them, they will. Few, indeed, will publicly acknowledge a state of feeling so unnatural; but there are some even of such. On the latter, all argument would, I fear, be utterly lost. Of the former, there may, be hope.

They tell us—and they are often sustained by those around them—that it is very inconvenient to be so confined to a child that they cannot leave home for a little while. Can it be their duty—for in these days, when virtue and religion, and everything good, are so highly complimented, no people are more ready to talk of *duty* than they who have the least regard to it—can it be their duty, they ask, to exclude themselves from the pleasures and comforts of social life for half or two thirds of their most active and happy years? Ought they not to go abroad, at least occasionally? But if so, and their children have no other source of dependence, must they not suffer? Is it not better, therefore, that they should be early accustomed to other food, for a part of the time? Besides, they may be sick; and then the child must rely on others; and will it not be useful to accustom it early to do so?

Perhaps few mothers are conscious that this train of reasoning passes through their minds. But that something like it is often made the occasion of substituting food which is less proper, for that furnished by Divine Providence, there cannot be a doubt. And the mischief is, that she who has gone so far, will not scruple, ere long, to go farther. And, strange and unnatural as it may seem, that mothers should turn over their children to be nursed wholly by others, in order to get rid of the inconvenience of nursing them at their own bosoms, it is only carrying out to its fullest extent, and reducing to practice, the train of reasoning mentioned above.

Nor is it necessary that I should stop here to denounce a course of conduct so unchristian and savage. I know it is very common in some countries; and those American mothers who ape the other eastern fashions, or countenance their sons and daughters in doing it, will not be slow to imitate this also—especially as it is a very *convenient* fashion. And I question whether I shall succeed in reasoning them out of it. Habit, both of thought and action, is exceedingly powerful. I will, therefore, confine myself chiefly to those efforts at prevention, from which much more is to be hoped, in the present state of society, than from direct attempts at cure.

It will be soon enough to leave a child with another person, when the mother is actually sick, or unavoidably absent; or when some other adequate cause is known to exist. We are to be governed, in these and similar cases, by general rules, and not by exceptions. The general rule, in the present case, is, that mothers can nurse their own children; and, if they have the proper disposition, that they can do it uninterruptedly.

But those who are so ready to become counsellors on these occasions, will tell us, perhaps, that the child must be "fed to spare the mother." That is to say, nursing weakens the mother, and the child must be taken away, a part of the time, to save her strength.

Now it may safely be doubted whether the process of nursing, in itself considered, does weaken, at all. The Author of nature has made provision for the secretion (formation) of the milk, whether the child receives it or not. If it is not taken by the child, or drawn off in some other way, one of two things must follow;—either it must be taken up by what are called absorbent vessels, and carried into the circulation, and chiefly thrown out of the system as waste matter, or it will prove a source of irritation, if not of inflammation, to the organs themselves which secrete it. In both cases, the strength of the mother is quite as likely to be taxed, as if the child received the milk in the way that nature intended.

Besides, on this very principle, the plan of saving a mother's strength by requiring another to nurse for her, is but saying that we will weaken one person to save another. Or if we feed the child, to "spare its mother,' what is this, in practice, but to say that the works of the Creator are very imperfect; and that he has thrown upon the mass of mankind a task to which they are not equal? For the mass of mankind are poor; and the poor, having neither the means nor the time to escape the duties in question, must submit to them, while their more wealthy neighbors escape.

But it is idle to defend customs so monstrous. They admit of no defence that has the slightest claim to solidity. The general rule then is, that mothers should nurse their own children.

## SEC. 2. *Conduct of the Mother.*

Originally it was not my intention to give directions, in this volume, in regard to the food, drink, &c., of the mother while nursing; but repeated solicitations on this point, have led me to the conclusion that a few general principles may be very properly introduced.

The future health, and even the moral well-being of the child, depend much more on the proper management of the mother herself than is usually supposed. How, indeed, can it be other wise? How can the mother's blood be constantly irritated with improper food and drink, without rendering the milk so? And how can a child draw, daily and hourly, from this feverish fountain, without being affected, not only in his physical frame, but in his very temper and feelings?

It is not enough that we adopt the principles already insisted on by some of our wisest medical men, and even by one or two medical societies, [Footnote: Those of Connecticut and New Hampshire.] that children in this way often acquire a propensity for exciting drinks, that may end in their downright intemperance. What if it should not, in every case, proceed quite so far as to make the child a drunkard? If it but lays the foundation of a constitutional fondness for *excitements,* it tends to disease. Indeed that, in itself, is a disease; and one, too, which is destroying more persons every year than the cholera, or even the consumption. Consumption has at most only slain her tens of thousands [Footnote: About 40,000 a year, in the United States, as nearly as it can be estimated.] a year; but a fondness for exciting food and drink—innocent and harmless as it is often supposed to be, and therefore only the more dangerous a foe—does not fail to slay every year, directly or indirectly, its hundreds of thousands. At least this is my own opinion.

Why, where can you find the individual who is not a slave to this perpetual rage within—this perpetual cry, "Who will show us any" physical "good"? Who, in this land of abundance, will eat or drink plain things? Who will eat simple bread, meat, potatoes, rice, pudding, apples, &c. or drink simple water? A few instances may be found, of late, in which people confine themselves to simple water for drink; but they are rather rare. And no wonder. They *must* be rare so long as an unnatural thirst is kept up everywhere by the most exciting and most strange mixtures of food. Where, I again ask, is the person who will eat and relish plain bread, plain meat, plain puddings, &c.? Certainly not in the nursery. No young mother—scarcely one I mean—will, for a single meal, confine herself to a piece of bread, the sweetest and best food in the whole world, unless it is hot, or toasted, or soaked, or buttered. A natural, healthy appetite, is as rare a thing on our planet, almost, as an inhabitant of the sun or moon.

I have seen more than one mother made sick by using, while nursing, improper food and drink. I have known milk punch, taken by stealth—(because how could the mother, it was said, ever have a supply of food for her poor child without it!)—to kindle a fever that came very near burning up the mother and child both. And yet, if I have once or twice succeeded in convincing the mother that she was only suffering the natural punishment of her own transgressions, I have never, so far as I now recollect, succeeded in making her believe that her iniquities were visited upon her unoffending infant.

There is everywhere the most painful apathy on this most painful subject. We see little children of all ages, everywhere, the victims of debility, and pain, and suffering, and disease and death, and yet we very seldom seem to search for one moment for the causes of this premature destruction. In fact most parents—even many intelligent mothers—at once stare, if you attempt to inquire into the causes of their child's death, as if it was either a kind of sacrilege, or an impeachment of their own parental affection. Diseases, even at this day, with the sun of science blazing in meridian splendor, they seem to regard as the judgments of heaven; and to think of tracing out the causes of the early death of half our race, is, in their estimation, not only idle, but wicked.

Yet this is obviously one of the first steps, every, where, which philanthropy demands; to say nothing of the demands of christianity. It is the first step for the physician, the first step for the educator, the first step for the parent, and above all, the mother. Nay; more—we must not suppress so great and important a truth—it is the first step for the legislator and the minister. What sense is there in continuing, century after century, and age after age, to expend all our efforts in merely *mending* the diseased half of mankind, when those same efforts are amply sufficient, if early and properly applied, not only to continue the lives of the whole, but to make them *whole beings*, instead of passing through life mere *fragments* of humanity?

But I must not forget that this is merely a small manual, not intended for those who make it their profession to teach the laws of God and man, but simply for young mothers. For the sake of erring humanity, would that I could, but for one moment, divest myself of the idea, that in writing for the young mother I am not writing for legislators and ministers! Would that I could banish from my mind the deep conviction that the mother is everywhere far more the law-giver to her infant—far more the arbiter of the present and eternal destiny of her child—than he who is more commonly regarded as such.

Every mother owes it, not only to herself—for on this part she is not *wholly* forgetful—but to her offspring, to abstain, during the period of nursing at least, from all causes which tend to produce a feverish state of her fluids. Among these are every form of premature exertion, whether in sitting up, laboring, conversing, or even thinking. It is of very great importance that both the body and the mind should be kept quiet; and the more so, the better.

Among the particular causes of fever to the young mother, Dr. Dewees enumerates spirits, wine, and other fermented liquors, a room too much heated, closed curtains, confined air, too much exposure, and too much company; and during the early period of confinement, broths and animal food.

There is nothing which he insists on more strongly, than the importance of fresh air. Indeed, the practice of confining a nursing woman in a space scarcely six feet square, and excluding the air surrounding her by curtains and closed windows, and subjecting her to the necessity of breathing twenty times the air that has already been as often discharged, filled with poison, from her lungs, is not too strongly reprobated by Dr. Dewees, or anybody else. But I have spoken of these things in the chapter which treats on "The Nursery." I would only observe, on this point, that if I were asked what one thing is most indispensable to the health of the nursing woman, I would reply, Fresh air; and if asked what were the second and third most important things, I would still repeat—in imitation of the orator of old, in regard to another subject—Fresh air, Fresh air.

This important ingredient in human happiness, and especially in the happiness of the young mother and her tender infant, can usually be had within doors, if pains enough be taken. But if the weather is fine and in every respect favorable, a woman who is in tolerable health may venture abroad a little in about three weeks after her confinement, and sometimes even in two. Whether her exercise be without or within doors, however, she should be effectually protected against chills, and against the influence of currents of cold air.

It has been incidentally stated, that Dr. Dewees objects to the mother's use, during her early period of nursing, of broths and animal food. This is about as much as we could reasonably expect from one who belongs to a profession whose members are, almost without exception, enslaved to the practice of flesh-eating. But even this advice of his, if duly followed, would be a great advance upon the practice which generally prevails. There is so universal a belief among females that they demand, at this period of their existence, not only a larger quantity of food than usual, but also that which is more stimulating in its quality, as almost to forbid the hopes of making much impression upon their minds. Many young mothers seem to consider themselves as licensed, during a part of their lives, not only to eat immoderately, and even to gluttony, but also to swallow almost every species of vile trash which a vile world affords.

How long will it be, ere the mother can be induced to take as much pains to select the most appropriate and most healthy aliment for herself and her child, as she now does that which is demanded by a capricious appetite, without the smallest reference to fitness or digestibility! How long will it be ere the mother can be brought to believe and feel that, in every step she takes, she is forming the habitation of an immortal spirit—a spirit, too, whose character and destiny, both present and eternal, must depend, in no small degree, upon the character of the dwelling it occupies while passing through this stage of earthly existence! How long will it be, before mothers can be made to believe even these two simple truths, that the nourishment, which the human being actually receives, is not always in exact proportion to the quantity of nutritious food which he throws into his stomach, and that the diet is always best for both mother and child, which is least exciting.

The Charleston Board of Health, during the existence of cholera in that city in 1836, publicly announced that the "best food is the least exciting," and this great truth is just as true in all other places and circumstances on the globe as it was then in South Carolina. And though I am far from believing that health depends more on food and drink than on all other things put together, as many seem to suppose, yet I am entirely of opinion that he who should devote himself successfully to the work of applying this truth, in all its bearings, to the dietetic practice of all mankind, would do more for their reformation—yes, and their salvation too—than has yet been done by any merely *human* being, since the first day of the creation.

## SEC. 3. *Nursing—how often.*

Many lay it down, as an invariable rule, that no system can be pursued with a child till it is six months old; and it must be admitted by all, that for several months after birth there are serious difficulties in the way of determining, with any degree of precision, how often a child should be nursed or fed. Still, there are a few rules of universal application; some of which are here presented.

1. A child should never be nursed, merely to quiet it; for if this be done, it will soon learn to cry, whenever it feels the slightest uneasiness, not only from hunger, but from other causes; merely to be gratified with nursing. Besides, if its cries should happen to be from illness, it is ten to one but the reception of anything into the stomach will do harm instead of good.

2. The stomach, like every other organ in the body which is muscular, must have time for rest; and this in the case of children as well as adults. But to nurse them too frequently is in opposition to this rule, and therefore of evil tendency.

3. For reasons which may be seen by the last rule, there should be regular seasons for nursing, and these should be adhered to, especially by night. When very young, once in three hours may not be too frequent; I believe that it is seldom proper to nurse a child more frequently than this. But whenever three hours becomes a suitable period by day, once in four hours will be often enough by night. I will not undertake to say at what precise age children should be nursed at intervals of three and four hours each; because some children are older, *constitutionally*, at three months, than others are at four.

There is one grand mistake, however, against which I must caution young mothers; which is, not to indulge the vain expectation that feeble infants will become robust, in proportion to their indulgence. On the contrary, it is the more necessary to be strict with feeble children, *because* they are feeble. To keep them hanging at the breast to invigorate them, is the very way to counteract our own intentions, and defeat our own purpose. Seasons of entire rest are even more important to their stomachs than to those of other persons.

4. But in order to secure intervals of rest, both to the strong and the feeble, we must avoid the pernicious habit of giving infants pap, and other delicacies, "between meals." Many a child's health is ruined by this practice. Nothing should be put into their stomachs for many months—if they are in health—but the mother's milk.

"This," says Dr. Dunglison, "is the sole food of the infant, and is consequently sufficiently nutrient to maintain life, and to minister to the growth, during the earliest periods of existence." [Footnote: Elements of Hygiene, page 271.] In another place, he says, "Milk is an appropriate nourishment at all ages, and is more so the nearer to birth."

## SEC. 4. *Quantity of Food.*

"We all know," says Dr. Dewees, "how easily the stomach may be made to demand more food than is absolutely required; first, by the repetition of aliment, and secondly, by its variety;—therefore both of these causes must be avoided. The stomach, like every other part, can, and unfortunately does, acquire habits highly injurious to itself; and that of demanding an unnecessary quantity of aliment is not one of the least. It should, therefore, be constantly borne in mind, that it is not the quantity of food taken into the stomach, that is available to the proper purposes of the system; but the quantity which can be digested, and converted into nourishment fit to be applied to such purposes."

There is a great deal of truth in these remarks; and especially in the closing one, that not all which is taken into the stomach is digested. It is highly probable, that the least quantity which is usually given to an infant is more than sufficient for the purposes of digestion; and that nearly every child in the arms of its mother, is over-fed.

I know it has been said, by some physicians—and by those who are sensible men, in other respects, too—that the child's stomach is a pretty correct guide in regard to quantity. If we give it too much, say they, it will reject it;—as if that were an end of the matter.

But it is not so. It is by no means harmless to fill the child's stomach as full as is possible without overflowing. Such a process, though it should not create disease directly, would produce a gluttonous habit. The stomach, being muscular, may be increased in size by use, like all other muscular organs. The hands, the arms, the legs, the feet, the fleshy portions of the face, even, may be disproportionally enlarged by constant use. Thus a sailor, who uses his hands and arms much more than his legs and feet, has the former unusually large; one who is much accustomed to walking, has large feet; and in a tailor, who from childhood uses his lower limbs comparatively little, they are both small and slender. On the same principle, the stomach, by inordinate use, and by carrying unreasonable loads, may be made nearly twice as large as nature intended, and may demand twice as much food. And I have no doubt that the bulk of mankind, young and old, eat about twice as much as nature, unperverted, would require.

If the suggestions of our last section are duly attended to, one of the causes which lead the stomach to demand an unreasonable quantity of food will be avoided—I mean the too frequent "repetition of aliment." And if we never depart from the general rule, already laid down, not to give the infant anything but its mother's milk, we shall escape the evils incident to variety.

### SEC. 5. *How long should milk be the only food.*

On this point, there is a great diversity of opinion. Perhaps the most approved role, of universal application, is, that the first change should be made in the child's diet, when the teeth begin to appear.

This period, it is well known, cannot be fixed to any particular age, but varies from the fifth to the twelfth month.

Some mothers, who have borne with me patiently to this place, will probably here object. "What child," they will ask, "would ever have any strength, brought up so?" Not only a little pap and gruel is, in their estimation, necessary, long before this period, but even many choice bits of meat.

Now I am very sure, that these choice bits—whatever they may be—given to a child before it has teeth, not only do no good, but actually do mischief. Indeed, that which does no good in the stomach must do harm, of course; since it is not only in the way, but acts like a foreign body there, producing more or less of irritation.

I ought to state, in this place, that many people—mothers among the rest—have very inadequate ideas of digestion. They appear to have no farther notion of the digestive process than that it consists in reducing to a pulp the substances which are swallowed; and hence, whatever is reduced to a pulp, they regard as being digested. Whereas nothing is better known to the anatomist and physiologist, than that this—the formation of *chyme* in the stomach—constitutes only a very small part of the digestive process. The chyme must pass into the duodenum and other portions of intestine beyond the stomach, and be retained there for some time, before it will form perfect chyle.

This is a more important part of the work of digestion than even the former. For, suppose the chyme to be perfect, though even this may be mere pulp, rather than chyme, and suppose it pass quietly along into the duodenum and other small intestines. All this process, thus far, may go on naturally enough, and yet the chyle may not be well formed, and the chymous mass may find its way out of the system without answering any of the purposes of nutrition. For no matter how well the food is dissolved in the stomach, if it do not become good and proper chyle, the blood which is formed will not be good and perfect blood; or, lastly, if it *seem* to make good blood, it may still be faulty, so that the particles which should be applied to build up or repair the system, are either not used, or if used, answer the purpose but imperfectly.

We hence see how little prepared a large proportion of the community, are, to judge of the digestibility or fitness of a substance for infants, by their own observation and experience merely; and how much more wisely they act, in contenting themselves with giving them—at least until they have teeth—such food only as the Author of nature seems to have assigned them;

especially when thus course, is precisely that which is recommended or sanctioned by nearly every judicious physician, as well as by almost all our writers on health.

### SEC. 6. *On Feeding before Teething.*

Having laid down the general rule, that until the appearance of teeth, the sole food of an infant should be the milk of its own mother, I proceed to speak of some of the more common exceptions to it.

EXCEPTION 1.—The first of these is when the supply furnished by the mother is scanty. There may be two causes of the scantiness of this supply; 1st, the want of suitable nourishment by the mother; and, 2dly, a feeble constitution, or bad health. In the former case, it should be her first object, as it undoubtedly will be that of her physician, to improve the quality of her diet; and in the latter, to restore her health, or at least invigorate her constitution.

In regard to the proper diet of a *mother*, as such, as well as the general management which her case requires, a volume might be written without exhausting the subject. But I have already said as much on this subject, in another place, as my limits will permit.

But we cannot wait for the mother's health to improve, and allow the infant to suffer, in the mean time, for a due supply of food. The appropriate question now is, How shall such a supply be furnished?

This should be done by means of an article resembling in its properties, as closely as possible, the mother's milk. For this purpose, we have only to mix with a suitable quantity of new cow's milk, one third of water, and sweeten it a little with loaf sugar. This is to be given to the child, at suitable intervals, and in proper quantities, by means of a common sucking bottle. It is, indeed, sometimes given with the spoon; but the bottle is better.

To the question, whether the child should be confined to this, till the period of weaning, Dr. Dewees answers, No. I am surprised at this; and my surprise is increased, when I find him, almost in the very next breath, urging with all his might, numerous reasons against the very common notion, that children in early life require a variety of food. He even insists on the importance of confining the child to a single article of food when it is practicable. Yet he has not given us so much as one reason why it is not practicable in the case before us; but has gone on to speak of barley water, gum arabic water, rice water, arrowroot, &c. I venture, therefore, to dissent from him, and to answer the foregoing question in the affirmative. When one good and substantial reason can be given for *change*, the decision will, however, be reconsidered.

I have already stated the general rule for preparing this substitute for the mother's milk. But there are several minor directions, which may be useful to those who are wholly without experience on the subject.

If possible, the milk used should not only be just taken from the cow, but should always be from the *same* cow; for it is well known, that the quality of milk often differs very materially, even among cows feeding in the same pasture, or from the same pile of hay; and the stomach becomes most easily reconciled to the mixture when it is uniform in its qualities. Great care should also be taken to see that the cow whose milk is used is young and healthy.

The mixture should not be prepared any faster than it is wanted, and should always be prepared in vessels perfectly clean and sweet, and given as soon as possible after it is prepared, to prevent any degree of fermentation. It is never so well to heat it by the fire. If taken from the cow just before it is used, and if the water to be added is warm enough, the temperature will hardly need to be raised any higher.

When it is impracticable, in all cases, to take milk for this purpose immediately from the cow, it should be kept, in winter, where it will not freeze; and in summer, where there will be no tendency to acidity.

Some mothers and nurses are addicted to the practice of passing the food through their own mouths, before they give it to the child—with a view, no doubt, to see that it is at a proper temperature. This practice is not only wholly unnecessary, but altogether disgusting, and even ridiculous. A thermometer would answer every purpose; and save even the trouble of another disgusting practice—that of blowing it with the breath.

The most proper season for giving the child this preparation, is immediately after it has been nursing. It is better for both mother and child, that the latter should nurse just as often as though the supply of food was adequate to his wants. And when his first supply is exhausted, then let him make up his meal from the sucking bottle. The great advantage of this plan is, that he will not be so likely in this way to be over-fed. If he is really needy, he will accept the bottle, even if he do not like it quite so well; if he refuse it, let him go without till he is hungry enough to receive it.

In regard to the water used in the preparation, only one thing needs to be said; which is, that it should be pure. If it is not, it should by all means be boiled. The sugar used should be of the very best kind; and the quantity not large; since if the preparation be too sweet, it readily becomes acid in the stomach.

There has been, and still is, a controversy going on among medical men, whether sugar is or is not hurtful to the young. "Who shall decide, when doctors disagree?" has often been asked. Without undertaking the task myself, I may perhaps be permitted to say, that I cannot see any reason why a substance so pure, and so highly nutritious as sugar—if given in very small quantity only—should prove injurious: though I do not regard the reasoning of Dr. Dewees as very conclusive on the subject, when, in reply to Dr. Cadogan, he has the following language—"If sugar be improper, why does it so largely enter into the composition of the early food of all animals? It is in vain that physicians declaim against this article, since it forms between seven and eight per cent of the mother's milk."—Now with me, the fact that milk and almost all other kinds of food are furnished with a measure of this substance, is the strongest reason I am acquainted with for making no additions. I believe, however, that they may sometimes be made, but not for these reasons.

EXCEPTION 2.—The second striking exception to the general rule that has been laid down, is when the mother is unable to nurse her own child from positive ill health, or when circumstances exist which render it obviously improper that she should do it. The following are some of the circumstances which render such a departure from nature indispensable.

1. When the mother is affected strongly with a hereditary disease, such as consumption or scrofula; or when her constitution is tainted, as it were, with venereal disease, or other permanent affections.

2. When nursing produces, uniformly, some very troublesome or dangerous disease in the mother; as cough, colic, &c.

3. There are a few instances in which the milk of the mother, owing to an unknown cause, has been found by experience to disagree with the child. In these circumstances, it is the unquestionable duty of the mother to resort wholly to feeding.

4. Sometimes the milk, at first abundant, fails suddenly, owing to some accidental or constitutional defect; and this failure becomes habitual. In all these circumstances, the proper resort is to a sucking bottle, or a hired nurse. I generally prefer the latter. The cases which seem to me to admit of the former, will be pointed out in the next section.

"When the bottle is used," says Dr. Dewees, "much care is requisite to preserve it sweet and free from all impurities, or the remains of the former food, by which the present may be rendered impure or sour; for which purpose a great deal of caution must be observed."

The business of feeding a child, whether by the bottle or the spoon, should never be hurried: the slower it is, the better. We should stop from time to time, during the process. Nor should the nourishment be given while lying down; it is much more pleasant, as well as more safe, to sit up.

A few thoughts more on the character and condition of the milk which we give to the young, will conclude the second division of this section.

Some are fond of boiling milk for infants; but to this I am decidedly opposed, so long as they are in health. Boiling takes away, or appears to take away, some of the best properties of the milk.

It is true that milk which is boiled does not turn sour so readily in hot weather; but it is quite unnecessary to boil milk in the common manner in order to present its changing, since such a result can be prevented by another process. You have only to put your milk in a kettle, cover it closely, and heat it quickly to the boiling point, and then remove and cool it as speedily as possible. This plan prevents the rising to the surface of that coat or pellicle which contains some of the most valuable properties of the milk.

I have already said that it was as necessary that the stomach should have rest as any other muscular organ. Some writers say that the infant should be kept perfectly quiet, at least half an hour, after each meal. This is certainly necessary with feeble children, but I question its necessity in the case of those who are strong and robust. I would not recommend, however, nor even tolerate, for one moment, the absurd practice of *jolting*, so common with a few ignorant nurses and, mothers, as if they could jolt down the food in the stomach with just as much safety as they can shake down the contents of a farmer's bag of produce. Such mothers as these should go and reside among the native tribes of Indians in Guiana, in South America, where they make it a point not only to stuff their children's stomachs as long as they will hold, but actually to shake it down.

Little less absurd than jolting is the custom of tossing a child high, in quick succession, which is practised not only after meals, but at other times. But on this point, I have treated elsewhere.

Some give the sucking bottle to children as a plaything. This is just about as wise a practice as that of giving them books as playthings. Both are done, usually, to save the time and trouble of those whose office it is to devote their time to the very purpose of managing and educating their offspring. The evil, however, of suffering the child to have the bottle when it pleases is, that he will thus be tasting food so often as to interfere with and disturb the process of digestion, to his great and lasting injury. For in this way, a part of the food will pass from the stomach into the bowels unchanged, or at least but imperfectly digested, where it is liable to become sour, and cause disease. It is not to be doubted that many diarrhoeas, as well as, other bowel affections, are produced in this way. Children that are always eating are seldom healthy; and we may hence see the reason.

In speaking of the importance of keeping the bottle, from which a child takes his food, perfectly clean and sweet, I ought to have extended the injunction much farther. There is a degree of slovenliness sometimes observable in those who manage children, both when they are sick and when they are in health, which even common sense cannot and ought not to tolerate. Every vessel which is used in preparing or administering anything for children, ought, after we have used it, to be immediately and effectually cleansed. How shocking is it to see dirty vessels standing in the nursery from hour to hour, becoming sour or impure! How much more so still, to see food in copper vessels, or in the red earthen ones, glazed with a poisonous oxyd! I speak now more particularly of vessels in which food is given; for with the administration of medicine, and nursing the sick, I do not intend in this volume to interfere.

EXCEPTION 3.—We come now to the consideration of those cases—for such it will not be doubted there are—where a hired nurse is to be preferred to feeding by the hand.

Before proceeding farther, however, it is important to say, that if a nurse could always be procured whose health, and temper, and habits were good, who had no infant of her own, and who would do as well for the infant, in every respect, as his own mother, it would be preferable to have no feeding by the hand at all.

But such nurses are very scarce. Their temper, or habits, or general health, will often be such as no genuine parent would desire, and such as they ought to be sorry to see engrafted, in any degree, on the child. For even admitting what is claimed by some, that the temper of the nurse does *not* affect the properties of the milk, and thus injure the child both physically and morally, still much injury may and inevitably will result from the influence of her constant presence and example.

Others have infants of their own, in which case either their own child or the adopted one will suffer; and in a majority of cases, it can scarcely be doubted *which* it will be. And I doubt the morality of requiring a nurse, in these cases, to give up her own child wholly. If *one* must be fed, why not our own, as well as that of another?

The only cases, then, which seem to me to justify the employment of a nurse, are where she possesses at least the qualifications above mentioned; and as these are rare, not many nurses, of course, would on this principle be employed. But when employed, it is highly desirable that the following rules should be observed:

1: The nurse should suckle the child at both breasts; otherwise he is liable to acquire a degree of crookedness in his form. There is another evil which sometimes results from the too common neglect of this rule, which is, that it endangers the deterioration of the quality of the milk.

2. The milk which is thus substituted for that of the mother, should be as nearly as possible of the same age as the child who is to receive it. It should be remembered, however, that the milk is not so good after the twelfth or thirteenth month, nor *quite* so good under the third.

3. When the parent or some trusty and confidential friend can, without the aid of interested spies and emissaries, have an eye to the general treatment, and especially to the moral management, it should be done; for even the best nurses may so differ in their principles, manners and habits from the parent, that the latter would deem it preferable to withdraw the child, and resort at once to feeding.

### SEC. 7. *From Teething to Weaning.*

This period will, of course, be longer or shorter according as the teeth begin to appear earlier or later, and according to the time when it is thought proper to wean.

On few points, perhaps, has there existed a greater diversity of opinion than in regard to the age most proper for weaning. The limits of this work do not permit a thorough discussion of the question; and I shall therefore be very brief in my remarks on the subject.

Dr. Cullen, whose opinion on topics of this kind is certainly entitled to much respect, thought that less than seven, or more than eleven months of nursing was injurious. Yet in some countries, and even in some parts of our own, the period is extended by the mother, from choice, to two years. And although the milk is not so good after the thirteenth or fourteenth month, I have never either known or heard that any evil consequences followed from the practice.

Dr. Loudon, a recent writer, observes, that the period of nursing has a great influence over the numbers of mankind in various countries, as is evinced by numerous facts. He adduces proofs of this, position. Thus, he says, in China, where the population is excessive, and the inhuman practice of infanticide is common, they wean a child as soon as it can put its hand to its mouth. On the other hand, the Indians of North America do not wean their children until they are old and strong enough to run about: generally they are suckled for a period of more than two years.

He then enters into a physiological inquiry why it is that British mothers do not usually suckle their children longer than ten months. He seems—though he does not give us his precise opinion—to think that, in all ordinary cases, the period of nursing ought to be protracted to two or three years, and that perhaps it would be better still to extend it to four or five. His remarks are so excellent, and withal so curious, and their tendency so humane, that we venture to insert one or two of his paragraphs entire.

"Certain it is, that the milk does not diminish particularly at that time, (ten months,) so far as regards quantity; and from the health of children reared without spoon-meat beyond this time, it as certainly undergoes no change in its quality. Children are sometimes so old before weaning, as to be able to ask for the breast; and it has not been remarked that the health of mothers, thus suckling, was in any way worse than that of their neighbors. Altogether, then, it may be asserted, that a mother is likely to enjoy better health, and to be less liable to sickness and death during lactation, than during pregnancy.

"Many women believe, or affect to believe, that the weakness they labor under arises from some latent moral or physical cause; but this weakness is not attributed to lactation in the earlier months of suckling, because the mother then considers herself fulfilling a necessary duty, which her constitution, for so long, is well able to bear. So soon, however, as the period of lactation has passed over, as it is established by custom or fashion, she imagines she is exceeding the intentions of nature, and she forthwith concludes that the continuance of suckling is the cause of her uncomfortable sensations. This whim being entertained, the child is weaned, and too often becomes the victim of a most reprehensible delusion.

"Since nature has furnished the mother with milk for a longer period than custom demands, it is evident that some good purpose for the mother and child was intended in this arrangement. Had it been otherwise, the secretion of milk would stop at a definite time, in like manner as the period of gestation is definite. That a child, in comparison with the young of the lower animals, is so long unable to provide for itself, strongly tends to corroborate the proofs already advanced—that nature originally had in view a more protracted period for lactation than is now allowed.

"Some writers, following the laws of nature, as they interpreted them, fixed the period of weaning at fifteen months, when the infant has got its eight incisors and four canine teeth. There are well-authenticated instances of mothers having suckled their children for three, four, five, and even seven consecutive years; we ourselves have known cases of lactation being prolonged far three and for four years, with the happiest results."

It appears to me better, therefore, that the child should be nursed, in all ordinary cases, from twelve to fifteen months; and when there are no special objections, about two years. As the change, whenever it is made, and however gradual it may be, is an important one, in its effects on the stomach and bowels, it is better to wean a little earlier or a little later, than to do so just at the close of summer or beginning of autumn, at which season bowel complaints are most common, most severe, and most dangerous. It is sufficiently unfortunate that teething should commence just at this period; but when we add another cause of irregular action, which we can control, to one which we *cannot*, we act very unwisely.

I have already observed that we may begin to feed children when the teeth begin to appear. By this is not meant that we should do so while the system is under the irritation to which teething usually, or at least often, subjects it. But when this is over, and a few teeth have appeared, it is usually a proper time to commence our operations.

The first food given should be precisely of the kind which has been recommended for those children who are fed by the hand. The rules and restrictions by which we are to be guided, are the same, except in one point, which is, that in the case we are now considering, the child should be fed *between nursing*.

Let not parents be anxious about their healthy children under two years, who have a supply of good milk, either from the mother or from the cow. For those that are feeble, a physician may and ought to prescribe—not medicine, but appropriate food, drink, &c.

When the grinding teeth have cut through, if we have any doubts in regard to the nutritive qualities of the food we are giving, we may improve it by adding, instead of the one third of pure water, a similar quantity of gum arabic water, barley water, or rice water. Some use a little weak animal broth; but this is unnecessary, and I think, on the whole, injurious, except for purposes strictly medicinal.

This course is so simple, and so far removed from that which is generally adopted, that few mothers will probably be willing to pursue it with perseverance, especially when the teeth appear very late. Those who are, however, will be richly rewarded, in the end, in the advantages; which will accrue to the child's health, and the vigor it will ensure to his constitution.

## SEC. 8. *During the process of Weaning.*

It has already been shown that, in weaning, some regard should be had to the season of the year; and that the end of summer and beginning of fall are of all periods the most unfavorable. The best time, on every account, is in the spring—in March, April, May, or June; and the next best is during the months of October and November. But December, January and February are better than July, August and September.

Weaning should never be sudden. We may safely and properly call upon those who are addicted to snuff or opium taking, tobacco chewing, rum drinking, and other habits which are purely artificial, to break off—*to wean themselves*—suddenly; since *they* can do so with considerable safety, and will seldom have the courage or the perseverance to do it otherwise. But with the child, in regard to his food, such a course will not be advisable. If we regard his future health or happiness, he must be weaned gradually.

The first proper step will be to give the child a little larger quantity of the cow's milk and gum arabic mixture, between nursings, at the same time increasing very gradually the intervals of nursing. When the intervals become six hours distant from each other, it will be best to add a little good bread to the milk with which it is fed, about two or three times a day. Arrowroot jelly, if he can be made to relish it, will be highly useful; but if not, some boiled rice, into which a little arrowroot has been sprinkled while boiling, may be added to his milk.

It may be worth the attempt to excite an aversion in the child to nursing his mother, so that be will refuse to nurse, if possible, of his own accord. This aversion may be excited by such an application of aloes, or some other offensive substance, as will cause him to withdraw himself from the breast as soon as he tastes it.

A serious mistake is often made, in connection with weaning, in giving the child not only too much food, but that which is too solid, or too rich. This mistake has undoubtedly grown out of the belief that his feeble condition *requires* it; whereas the truth is, that he neither needs food at this period, nor is capable of digesting it. For let us be as judicious in the process of weaning as we may, the tone of the child's stomach will be somewhat reduced, or in other words, its powers of digestion will be weakened by it; and to give it strong food, or overload it with that which is weaker, is not only unreasonable and unphilosophical, but cruel. And if there should be a tendency in the child's constitution to rickets, scrofula, consumption, and other wasting diseases, such a course would be likely to bring them on, and destroy life.

"When milk will agree," says Dr. Dewees, "there is no food so proper. It may be employed in any of its combinations, with good wheaten bread, rice, sago, &c., only remembering that when either of these articles is found to agree, it should be continued perseveringly, until it may become offensive. In this case, some new combination may be required." I do not see the necessity of continuing one kind of food till it *offends*. Besides, I do not believe that these simple articles of food are apt to become offensive to stomachs that have not already been spoiled. But whether a single dish should or should not come to be offensive, I greatly prefer an occasional change.

Buchan, in his Advice to Mothers, has recommended it to them to boil bread for their infants, in water. It should not, for this purpose—nor indeed for any other—be new; it is best at one or two days, old. It may be boiled in a small quantity of water, or what is still better, of milk; or it may be steamed till it becomes soft and light, almost like new bread, but without any of the objectionable properties of that which is wholly new. To bread, thus prepared, is to be added a suitable quantity of milk, fresh from the cow, and a little diluted with water, but not boiled.

But as there may be, here and there, at any age, a stomach with which milk, with bread, or rice, or sago, will not agree—though I think they must be very rare cases—we may be allowed to substitute for it a solution of "gum arabic, in the proportion of an ounce to a pint of water," to which may be added a little sugar; and if the child is old enough to observe the color, just milk enough to change the appearance. Another preparation for the same purpose consists of rennet whey, a little sweetened, and "disguised, if necessary, as just stated."

The health of the mother, too, during the period of weaning, often needs great attention. Let her avoid medicine, however, if possible. A due regard to food, drink, exercise, and rest of body and mind, &c., will usually be found more effective, as well as more permanently efficacious.

## SEC. 9. *Food subsequently to Weaning.*

You will allow me to introduce in this place, some of the sentiments of Dr. Cadogan, an English physician, from a little work on the management of children. [Footnote: Though Dr. C.'s remarks will apply more closely to England in 1750, they are by no means inapplicable to the United States in 1837.] I do it with the more pleasure because, though he wrote almost a century ago, he urges the same general principles on which I have all along been insisting: hence it will be seen that mine are no new-fangled notions. His remarks refer to the young of every age, but chiefly to early infancy and childhood. It will be found necessary, in some instances, to abridge, but I shall endeavor not to misrepresent the Doctor's views.

"Look over the bills of mortality. Almost half of those who fill up that black list, die under five years of age; so that half the people that come into the world go out of it again, before they become of the least use to it or to themselves. To me, this seems to deserve serious consideration.

"It is ridiculous to charge it upon nature, and to suppose that infants are more subject to disease and death than grown persons; on the contrary, they bear pain and disease much better—fevers especially; and for the same reason that a twig is less hurt by a storm than an oak.

"In all the other productions of nature, we see the greatest vigor and luxuriancy of health, the nearer they are to the egg or bud. When was there a lamb, a bird, or a tree, that died because it was young? These are under the immediate nursing of unerring nature; and they thrive accordingly.

"Ought it not, therefore, to be the care of every nurse and every parent, not only to protect their nurslings from injury, but to be well assured that their own officious services be not the greatest evils the helpless creatures can suffer?

"In the lower class of mankind, especially in the country, disease and mortality are not so frequent, either among adults or their children. Health and posterity are the portion of the poor—I mean the laborious. The want of superfluity confines them more within the limits of nature; hence they enjoy the blessings they feel not, and are ignorant of their cause.

"In the course of my practice, I have had frequent occasion to be fully satisfied of this; and have often heard a mother anxiously say, 'the child has not been well ever since it has done puking and crying.'

"These complaints, though not attended to, point very plainly to the cause. Is it not very evident that when a child rids its stomach of its contents several times a day, it has been overloaded? While the natural strength lasts, (for every child is born with more health and strength than is generally imagined,) it cries at or rejects the superfluous load, and *thrives apace*; that is, grows very fat, bloated, and distended beyond measure, like a house lamb.

"But in time, the same oppressive cause continuing, the natural powers are overcome, being no longer able to throw off the unequal weight. The child, now unable to cry any more, languishes and is quiet.

"The misfortune is, that these complaints are not understood. The child is swaddled and crammed on, till, after gripes, purging, &c., it sinks under both burdens into a convulsion fit, and escapes farther torture. This would be the case with the lamb, were it not killed, when full fat.

"That the present mode of nursing is wrong, one would think needed no other proof than the frequent miscarriages attending it, the death of many, and the ill health of those that survive. But what I am going to complain of is, that children, in general, are over-clothed and over-fed, and fed and clothed improperly. To these causes I attribute almost all their diseases.

"But the feeding of children is much more important to them than their clothing. Let us consider what nature directs in the case. If we follow nature, instead of leading or driving her, we cannot err. In the business of nursing, as well as physic, art, if it do not exactly copy this original, is ever destructive.

"If I could prevail, no child should ever be crammed with any unnatural mixture, till the provision of nature was ready for it; nor afterwards fed with any ungenial diet whatever, at least for the *first three months*; for it is not well able to digest and assimilate other elements sooner.

"I have seen very healthy children that never ate or drank anything whatever but their mother's milk, for the first ten or twelve months. Nature seems to direct to this, by giving them no teeth till about that time. The call of nature should be waited for to feed them with anything more substantial; and the appetite ought ever to precede the food—not only with regard to the daily meals, but those changes of diet which opening, increasing life requires. But this is never done, in either case; which is one of the greatest mistakes of all nurses.

"When the child requires more solid sustenance, we are to inquire what and how much is most proper to give it. We may be well assured there is a great mistake either in the quantity or quality of children's food, or both, as it is usually given them, because they are made sick by it; for to this mistake I cannot help imputing nine in ten of all their diseases.

"As to quantity, there is a most ridiculous error in the common practice; for it is generally supposed that whenever a child cries, it wants victuals: it is accordingly fed ten or twelve or more times in a day and night. This is so obvious a misapprehension, that I am surprised it should ever prevail.

"If a child's wants and motions be diligently and judiciously attended to, it will be found that it never cries, but from pain. Now the first sensations of hunger are not attended with pain; accordingly, a very young child that is hungry will make a hundred other signs of its want, before it will cry for food. If it be healthy, and quite easy in its dress, it will hardly ever cry at all. Indeed, these signs and motions I speak of are but rarely observed, because it seldom happens that children are ever suffered to be hungry.[Footnote: That which we commonly observe in them, in such cases, and call by the name of hunger, the Doctor, I suppose would regard as morbid or unnatural feeling, wholly unworthy of the name of HUNGER.]

"In a few, very few, whom I have had the pleasure to see reasonably nursed, that were not fed above two or three times in twenty-four hours, and yet were perfectly healthy, active, and happy, I have seen these signals, which were as intelligible as if they had spoken.

"There are many faults in the quality of children's food.

"1. It is not simple enough. Their paps, panadas, gruels, &c. are generally enriched with sugar, spices, and other nice things, and sometimes a drop of wine—none of which they ought ever to take. Our bodies never want them; they are what luxury only has introduced, to the destruction of the health of mankind.

"2. It is not enough that their food should be simple; it should also be light. Many people, I find, are mistaken in their notions of what is light, and fancy that most kinds of pastry, puddings, custards, &c. are light; that is, light of digestion. But there is nothing heavier, in this sense, than unfermented flour and eggs, boiled hard, which are the chief ingredients in some of these preparations.

"What I mean by light food—to give the best idea I can of it—is, any substance that is easily separated, and soluble in warm water. Good bread is the lightest thing I know, and the fittest food for young children. Cows' milk is also simple and light, and very good for them; but it is often injudiciously prepared. It should never be boiled; for boiling alters the taste and properties of it, destroys its sweetness, and makes it thicker, heavier, and less fit to mix and assimilate with the blood."

---

It is hardly necessary for me to repeat, that in these general views of Dr. C., with a few exceptions, I entirely concur; indeed some of them have already been presented. But I have expressed my doubts of the soundness of his conclusion in regard to sugar. Used with food, in very small quantity, by persons whose stomachs are already in a good condition, both sugar and molasses, especially the former, appear to me not only harmless, but wholesome and useful.

On the subject of simplicity in children's food, I should be glad to enlarge. There is nothing more important in diet than simplicity, and yet I think there is nothing more rare. To suit the fashion, everything must be mixed and varied. I have no objection to variety at different meals, both for children and adults; indeed I am disposed to recommend it, as will be seen hereafter. But I am utterly opposed to any considerable variety at the same meal; and above all, in a single dish. The simpler a dish can be, the better.

But let us look, for a moment, at the dishes of food which are often presented, even at what are called plain tables.

Meats cannot be eaten—so many persons think—without being covered with mustard, or pepper, or gravy—or soaked in vinegar; and not a few regard them as insipid, unless several of these are combined. Few people think a piece of plain boiled or broiled muscle (lean flesh) with nothing on it but a little salt, is fit to be eaten. Everything, it is thought, must be rendered more stimulating, or acrid; or must be swimming in gravy, or melted fat or butter.

Bread, though proverbially the staff of life, can scarcely be eaten in its simple state. It must be buttered, or honied, or toasted, or soaked in milk, or dipped in gravy. Puddings must have cherries or fruits of some sort, or spices in them, and must be sweetened largely. Or perhaps—more ridiculous still—they must have suet in them. And after all this is done, who can eat them without the addition of sauce, or butter, or molasses, or cream? Potatoes, boiled, steamed or roasted, delightful as they are to an unperverted appetite, are yet thought by many people hardly palatable till they are mashed, and buttered or gravied; or perhaps soaked in vinegar. In short, the plainest and simplest article for the table is deemed nearly unfit for the stomach, till it has been buttered, and peppered, and spiced, and perhaps *pearlashed*. Even bread and milk must be filled with berries or fruits. Where can you find many adults who would relish a meal which should consist entirely of plain bread, without any addition; of plain potatoes, without anything on them except a little salt; of a plain rice pudding, and nothing with it; or of plain baked or boiled apples or pears? And *could* such persons be found, how many of them would bring up their children to live on such plain dishes?

It need not be wondered at, that a palate which has been so long tickled by variety, and by so many stimulating mixtures of food, should come to regard cold water for drink as insipid; and should feel dissatisfied with it, and desirous of boiling some narcotic or poisonous herb in it, or brewing it with something which will impart to it more or less of alcohol. The wonder is, not that some of our epicures become drunkards, but that all of them do not.

Dr. Cadogan alludes to a sad mistake everywhere made about *light* food; and condemns, very justly, hard-boiled custards, pastry, &c. It is very strange that these substances—for these are among the injurious articles which I call mixtures—should ever have obtained currency in the world, to the exclusion of bread, which, as the same writer justly says, is among the lightest articles of food which are known.

It is strange, in particular, what views people have about bread. Judging from what I see, I am compelled to believe that there are few who regard it in any other light than as a kind of necessary evil. They appear to eat it, not because they are fond of it, by itself, but because they *must* eat it; or rather, because it is a fashionable article; and not to make believe they eat it, at the least, would be unfashionable. They will get rid of it, however, when they can. And when they must eat it, they soak it, or cover it with butter or milk, or something else which will render it tolerable—or toast it. And use it as they may, it must be hot from the oven. After it is once cold, very few will eat it. The idea, above all, of making a full meal of simple cold bread, twenty-four hours old, would be rejected by ninety-nine persons in a hundred; and by some with abhorrence.

People not only dislike bread, but regard it as unnutritious. I have heard many a fond parent say to the child who ate no meat, and seemed to depend almost wholly on bread—"Why, my dear child, you will starve if you eat no meat. Do at least put some butter on your bread or your potatoes." A thousand times have I been admonished, when eating my vegetable dinner during the hot and fatiguing days of summer—for I was bred to the farm, and ate little or no meat till I was fourteen years of age—to eat more butter, or cheese, or something that would give me strength; for I could not work, they said, without something more nourishing than bread and the other vegetables. And yet few if any boys of my age did more work, or performed it better, or with more ease, than myself. And I early observed the same thing in other vegetable eaters.

The truth is, there is nothing in the world better adapted to the daily wants of the human stomach than good bread; and few things more nutritious. There may be a little more nutriment in eggs or jelly; but if the former are hard-boiled, the stomach cannot digest them; and fat meat of any kind is digested with great difficulty. Indeed it is doubtful whether stomachs in temperate climates digest fat at all. They may dissolve it, but that is not making good chyle of it. They may even reduce it to chyle; *but chyle is not blood*. Fat may slip through the system without much of it *adhering*; and I think it pretty evident that it usually does so.

The muscle—the lean part of animals—may be nearly as nutritious as good bread, and is more easily digested. But it is very far from being proved that, for the healthy, those things are always best which are most easily digested. Nobody will pretend that potatoes are better for us than bread; and yet the experiments of Dr. Beaumont seem to prove that boiled or roasted potatoes are much more quick and easy of digestion than bread of the first and best quality. Even over-boiled eggs and raw cabbage, bad as they are, are dissolved in the stomach, and appear to be digested as quick, if not quicker, than good wheat bread. But nobody in the world will pretend they form more wholesome food. Neither is meat—even *lean* meat—necessarily more wholesome, or better calculated to give strength than bread, simply be cause it is more quickly and easily digested. It would be nearer the truth to say, that those substances which digest slowest (provided they do not irritate) are best adapted to the wants of the human stomach.

The philosopher LOCKE—perhaps from his knowledge of medicine—gives some excellent directions on this subject. "Great care should be used," be says, that the child "eat bread plentifully, both alone and with everything else; and whatever he eats that is solid, make him chew it well." This writer, by the way, supposed that the teeth were made to be used in beating our food; and that we ought neither to swallow it without chewing, as is customary in our busy New England, nor to mash or soak it in order to save the labor of mastication—a practice almost equally universal. But let us hear his own words.

> "As for his diet, it ought to be very plain and simple; and if I might advise, flesh should be forborne, at least till he is two or three years old. But of whatever advantage this may be to his future health and strength, I fear it will hardly be consented to by parents, misled by the custom of eating too much flesh themselves, who will be apt to think their children—as they do themselves—in danger to be starved; if they have not flesh at least twice a day. This I am sure, children would breed their teeth with much less danger, be freer from diseases while they were little, and lay the foundations of a healthy and strong constitution much surer, if they were not crammed so much as they are, by fond mothers and foolish servants, and were kept wholly from flesh the first three or four years of their lives."

Were Locke still living, I should like to interrogate him at this place. He first speaks of giving children no meat till they are two or three years old; and then afterwards extends the period to three or four. The question I would put is this: If the child is healthier without meat till he is three or four years old, why not till he is thirteen or fourteen; or even till thirty, or forty, or seventy? And is not Professor Stuart, of Andover—a meat eater himself, and an advocate for its moderate use by those who have already been trained to the use of it—is not the Professor, I say, more than half right when he asserts, as I have heard him, that it may be well to train all children, from the first, to the exclusive use of vegetable food?

I have a few more extracts from Locke, particularly on the subject of bread.

> "I should think that a good piece of well made and well baked brown bread would be often the best breakfast for my young master. I am sure it is as wholesome, and will make him as strong a man, as greater delicacies; and if he be used to it, it will be as pleasant to him.
>
> "If he, at any time, call for victuals between meals, use him to nothing but dry bread. If he be hungry more than wanton, bread will go down; and if he be not hungry, it is not fit that he should eat. By this you will obtain two good effects. First, that by custom he will come to be in love with bread; for, as I said, our palates and stomachs, too, are pleased with the things we are used to. Another good you will gain hereby is, that you will not teach him to eat more nor oftener than nature requires.
>
> "I do not think that all people's appetites are alike; some have naturally stronger and some weaker stomachs. But this I think, that many are made gormands and gluttons by custom, that were not so by nature. And I see, in some countries, men as lusty and strong, that eat but two meals a day, as those that have set their stomachs, by a constant usage, to call on them for four or five.
>
> "The Romans usually fasted till supper, the only set meal, even of those who ate more than once in a day; and those who used breakfasts, as some did at eight, same at ten, others at twelve of the clock, and some later, neither ate flesh nor had anything made ready for them.
>
> "Augustus, when the greatest monarch on the earth, tells us he took a piece of dry bread in his chariot; and Seneca, in his 83d epistle, giving an account how be managed himself when he was old, and his age permitted indulgence, says that he used to eat a piece of dry bread for his dinner, without the formality of sitting to it. Yet Seneca, as it is well known, was wealthy.
>
> "The masters of the world were brought up with this spare diet, and the young gentlemen of Rome felt no want of strength or spirit because they ate but once a day. Or if it happened by chance that any one could not fast so long as till supper, their only set meal, he took nothing but a bit of dry bread, or at most a few raisins or some such slight thing with it, to stay his stomach. And more than one set meal a day was thought so monstrous that it was a reproach, as low as Caesar's time, to make an entertainment, or sit down to a table, till towards sunset. Therefore I judge it most convenient that my young master should have nothing

> but bread for breakfast. I impute a great part of our diseases in England to our eating too much flesh, and too little bread. Dry bread, though the best nourishment, has the least temptation."

I shall not undertake to defend all the sentiments of Mr. Locke in these extracts; but in regard to the main point—the nutritive properties and wholesome tendency of bread, and the importance of making it a principal article of diet for children—I think his views are just. In short, they do not differ, substantially, from those of a large proportion of the best writers on this subject in every country, during the last three hundred years. As if with one voice, they dissuade from the use of too much animal food for the young, and encourage the use of a larger proportion of vegetable food—bread, plain puddings, rice, potatoes, turnips, beets, apples, pears, &c., and milk.

Yet they all, or nearly all, seem to write just as if they did not expect to be believed; or if believed, to be followed. They seem to regard mankind as so inveterately attached to old habits, and so much addicted to flesh eating, that there is little hope of reclaiming them.

Now, though my opinions are no more entitled to respect than many of theirs, I hope for greater success than they appear to do. I expect that many young mothers who read this work, will be led to think and inquire further on the subject; and if they find that the views here advanced are in accordance with reason, and common sense, and higher authority, I am not without hope that they will reform, and do what they can to reform their neighbors.

I have dwelt the longer, in this section, on the *general* principles of diet, because I am of opinion that whatever is true, on this subject, in regard to the diet of children, soon after weaning, is equally, or nearly equally applicable to the whole of childhood, youth, manhood and age. It is not true that one period of life, and one mode of employment, demands a diet essentially different from that which is demanded at another period, and in other circumstances; provided always, that the individual is in health. Occasional instances of the kind, there may be; but they are not numerous.

The digestive powers of the young are more nearly as strong as those of the adult than is usually admitted, and they are much more active. They require a less quantity of food, undoubtedly; and they should be fed at shorter intervals. But as a general rule, what is best for them, as regards its quality, at three years old, is best for them at thirty; or, should they live so long, at ninety. I repeat it; there is very little difference in the nature of the food required ever after teething.

Let me not be understood as saying that the strong, and the robust, and the active cannot digest food which the weak, and enervated, and indolent cannot. Undoubtedly they can. But this does not prove that they *ought* to do it. It does not prove that their strength and vigor were not given them for other purposes than to be expended on the poorer substances for food, when they might have better. Nor is it true, as often pretended, that the hard laborer needs either more food, or that which is of a stronger quality, just in proportion to the severity of his labor. The man or the child who labors moderately, just sufficient for the purposes of health, and labors with his hands in the open air, needs rather *more* food than the indolent or the sedentary, or those who labor to excess; but not that which is of a stronger quality. It is he who labors to excess—if any difference of quality were required at all—who should eat milder food, as well as less in quantity.

Some physicians there are who tell us that all mankind would live longer, as well as be more healthful, if they ate nothing but bread, and drank nothing but water. It may be so, but I do not believe it. Water, as I shall show hereafter, is indeed the only appropriate drink; but I do not believe that bread, even after the second year, is in all cases and circumstances the best food. Besides that the experiments of Majendie and other physiologists go a little way—though not far, I confess—to prove that animals generally, (and if so, why not man, as well as the rest?) thrive best with some degree of variety in their food, it seems to me more in accordance with the general intentions of the Creator, so far as we can discover what they are.

While, therefore, I deny that either milk or bread is better, in all cases, for human sustenance, than any other articles of food, I must, at the same time, be permitted to regard them as among the best, and as deserving more general attention. Every infant, after leaving the breast, should, as it seems to me, make bread, in some of its forms, a chief article of food.

This article, so justly and emphatically called the staff of life, may be found in almost every country. Common sense seems to have dictated the propriety of its use; though fashion has often led us to overlook or despise it—like air, and fire, and water, and nearly every other common but indispensable blessing.

The best kind of bread is made from wheat, the worst from bark, sawdust, &c. Wood and bark afford so little nutriment, that it is only in such countries as Norway, Sweden, Lapland. Iceland, Greenland, and Siberia, that the inhabitants can be induced to make use of them. Here they are often useful; either because people cannot get food which is better, or to blend with their fat or oily animal food. For it should never be forgotten, that healthy digestion requires a large proportion of innutritious matter along with the pure nutriment. In order to make bread from wheat, the meal should not be bolted. If it seems to contain particles which are too coarse, it may be well to pass it through a coarse family sieve; but the best bread I have ever eaten, as well as the cleanest and neatest, was not sifted at all.

I know there is an almost universal prejudice against this sort of bread. Some complain that it scratches their throats; others, that it is tasteless; and others still, that it does not agree with them. With others there is another objection—which is that bread of this sort has sometimes been called *dyspepsia* bread; and with others still, that it has been called *Graham* bread. Either of these appellations seems sufficient to condemn it.

Now as to the harshness, this is owing to its being made of bad materials, or to its being baked too hard, or kept too long. Much of what they call dyspepsia bread, in our cities, is evidently made by mixing the bran and flour of wheat after they have been once separated; besides which, in not a few cases, the finest of the flour appears to be taken away. Now bread made of such materials thus combined, will always be darker colored, as well as harsher, than when made from the wheat, simply ground without any bolting, and wet up in the usual manner. Such bread is best two or three days old. After four days, it becomes dry and somewhat harsh.

They who complain that such bread is insipid, are persons whose appetites have been injured by food which is high-seasoned; and who, if they eat bread at all, must eat it hot, or soaked in butter. No wonder such persons do not like plain bread, and say it is tasteless. But it must not be denied that bakers often suffer this kind of bread to be over-risen, in order to make it sufficiently light and porous. This renders it less tasteful, and from the saleratus they use, less wholesome.

No child who has been accustomed, from the first, to good wheaten bread, made of unbolted meal, and not less than one day old, will ever prefer any other, until he has been rendered capricious on this subject, and wishes to change for the sake of changing, or until he has been misled by surrounding example. I speak from observation when I say that infants, whose habits have not been depraved, will not prefer hot bread of any kind. "It is hot, mother," I have heard them say, as an apology for refusing a piece of bread; but never, "It is cold," or "It is too old."

It is the epicurean—it is he with whom it is a sufficient objection to any kind of food whatever, that he has used it for several successive meals or days—that is most ready to complain of good bread. He whose habits are correct, and who is the more unwilling to change any of his articles of diet, the longer he has been in the use of them, and who only changes them, or uses variety, from principle—he, I say, will never complain of harshness or want of taste in good wheat bread; nor will it be an objection of weight with him that *Mr. Graham* has recommended it, or that it has either prevented or cured *dyspepsia*.

Nor will the epicurean himself complain that bread is insipid, after being confined to it for a month or six weeks. He will then find a sweetness in it, for which he had long sought in vain in the more delicate and costly viands of a luxurious, and expensive, and unchristian modern table.

It is they only who observe simplicity, and confine themselves to very plain food, who truly enjoy pleasure in eating. The bulk of mankind benumb their sense of taste by their high-seasoned, over-stimulating food and drink, and by such constant variety and strange mixtures; and thus, in their eager cry, "Who will show us any good?" they actually enjoy less than he who eats plain food, and is contented with it.

Bread of all kinds is greatly improved in whiteness and pleasantness by being wet with milk; though even when wet with nothing but water, there is a solid and rational sweetness to it, of which the despisers of bread, and devourers of much flesh and condiments never dreamed, and never will dream, till they reform their habits.

If children are furnished with good bread, on the plan of Mr. Locke, there is no doubt that they will relish it most keenly; that their attachment to it will strengthen, and that unless we give them other food occasionally, from principle, or seduce them by depraving their tastes, they will continue it through life. "Train up a child in the way he should go, and when he is old he will not depart from it," is a general rule, and has as few exceptions, when applied to the diet of a child, as when it is applied to his moral tastes and preferences.

With those parents who, though convinced of the justness of the views here advanced, have already trained their children in the way they should *not* go, but are anxious to retrace their steps as far as possible, there will here be a difficulty. "Our children," they will say, "do not, at present, *relish* the kind of bread you speak of; and how shall we bring them to do so? or is the thing indeed possible?"

The answer to these inquiries is easy. Such parents have only to confine their children to the kinds of food which they deem proper for them, a few weeks or a few months, and they will soon relish them. If those who are old enough to be convinced can be brought to unite heartily in the change, and to endeavor to be pleased with it, the work of reformation will be more pleasant and probably more speedy. I have never found any difficulty of bringing myself to relish in a very short time an article of food for which I had no relish before, and to which I had even a dislike, provided I was thoroughly convinced it was best for me, and was earnest in the desire of change—except sweet oil, to which I was about six months in becoming reconciled.

It is with physical, as with moral habits, in their formation. We should fix on what we believe, from experience, observation, and divine and human testimony, is best for us, and habit will soon render it agreeable. It is important, even to health, that food should be agreeable; but as I have already said, what we know to be best for us will soon become agreeable, if we confine ourselves to it; and to our children also, if we confine them to it, in like manner.

Next to bread made of wheat—when that cannot be procured—is a mixture of wheat and Indian meal; but the proportion of the latter should be the smallest. Wheat, rye, and Indian, in the proportion of one third of each, make excellent bread, sometimes called *third* bread. Rye and Indian make a tolerable bread. Rye alone is not so good. The want, in the latter, of the vegetable principle called gluten, makes its general use of very questionable propriety.

Indian meal alone, baked in cakes by the fire, if eaten only in small quantities, is a very nutritious and by no means unwholesome bread. But its sweetness, and the general fondness which people who are accustomed to its use have for it, lead them to eat it in too large proportions, if they use it while it is warm. In these circumstances, it proves itself too active for the stomach and bowels. If warm, six ounces is as much as a hearty adult ought to eat of it at once; and children should of course take much less. It is less active on the bowels, and scarcely less agreeable, as soon as we become accustomed to it, if eaten when it is cold—even if baked in loaves, in the oven.

Potatoes, added to unbolted wheat flour, make excellent bread; and so, as I am informed, does rice. Of the latter, however, I have never eaten. Oats and barley, and many other grains and substances, will make bread; but it is of an inferior kind.

The question may again recur, after this extended series of remarks, whether I intend to confine the young almost exclusively to bread, in one or another of its forms. We shall see how this is, presently.

While bread, therefore, should constitute a part, at least, and sometimes the whole of a meal, a great variety of other articles are not only admissible, but desirable. Among these may be mentioned plain puddings.

One of the most wholesome puddings is made of Indian meal, enclosed in a bag and boiled. Nearly allied to this is the common hasty pudding; but the last is less wholesome, because it requires less chewing; and it ought to have been observed, before now, that after weaning, any food is digested better which has undergone the process of thorough mastication.

Boiled rice, though hardly to be regarded as a pudding, is very nutritious, and very easy of digestion. I am not without doubts, however, in regard to the utility of a large proportion of rice, as food. A dinner of it, two or three times a week, I believe to be wholesome; but used too frequently, it seems to me not active enough for the stomach and bowels; having in this respect precisely a contrary effect to that of warm Indian cakes. The common notion that rice has a tendency to make people blind, is entirely unfounded. Its worst effect is when eaten without being boiled through. In such cases, I have known it to do mischief; perhaps because it was swallowed without much chewing. Some grind it, and use the flour; but I cannot recommend it to be used in this manner.

The best pudding in the world is a loaf of bread, (What!—you will say—bread again?) three or four or five days old, boiled, or rather *steamed*, in milk. All kinds of bread are excellent for this purpose, but wheat and Indian are the best. They are excellent even without milk—that is, simply steamed.

Puddings made of the flour of wheat, rye, buckwheat, &c., are less wholesome than those which have been already mentioned. And all sorts of puddings are less wholesome, when eaten as hot as our unreasonable fashions require, than when their temperature is quite below that of our bodies. I would not have them so cold as to chill us, for this would be to go to the other, though less dangerous extreme; but they ought to be cool. Too much heat is an unnatural stimulus, likely to leave more or less debility behind it. In addition to this, those who eat hot food are more exposed to take cold, in consequence of it.

With none of these puddings ought we to mix any fruits, green or dried—not even raisins. Some of the more important properties of nearly every kind of fruit or berry are lost by boiling, unless we eat the water in which they are boiled, and save the vapor which would otherwise escape. I am not in favor of boiled fruit generally, especially if boiled in puddings.

Puddings, like most other kinds of food—even bread—may be slightly salted: not that this is indispensable, but because the balance of human testimony is in its favor. The argument that we evidently need salt because the other animals require it, is without much weight. The other animals do not *generally* require or use it.[Footnote: Some considerable savage nations use no salt, and a few have a strong aversion to it.] The cases so often triumphantly mentioned, where animals appear to thrive better from the use of it, are only exceptions to the general rule, nor are they very numerous in comparison with the whole race of animals. Still I have no objections to its moderate use. It may be useful in preventing worms; though there are doubts even of that. In large quantities, it is unquestionably hurtful.

But neither fruits nor berries—permit me to repeat the sentiment—no, nor any such thing as cinnamon or spices, nor even sugar or molasses in any considerable quantity, should go into the composition of any sort of pudding. If the puddings are not sweet enough without, it is better to add a little sugar or molasses on your plate. Nor should sauces, or cream, or butter, or suet be used in or upon them; though of all these substances, cream is least injurious. Nutmegs, grated cheese, &c., are unnecessary and hurtful. Cheese should never be eaten, in any way.

There is one thing, however, which may be eaten in moderate quantity with all sorts of puddings and with bread; I mean milk. I say eaten *with*, for it is better never to put these substances, nor indeed any other, *into* the milk. The bread, pudding, &c., should be eaten by itself, and the milk by itself, also. In this way we shall not be liable to cheat the teeth out of what is justly their due, and then make the deranged stomach and general system pay for it.

Potatoes are a good article of diet—to be used once a day—though they are not very nutritious. They are best either steamed or roasted in the ashes. They are also excellent when boiled. Turnips are also good. Onions are not so useful as is generally supposed, except for the purposes of medicine.

Beets; in small quantity, and carrots and asparagus, and above all, beans and peas—but not their pods—are tolerable food once a day, during most of the year, except it be the middle of the winter. But neither these, nor potatoes, nor any other vegetables, ought to be cooked in any way with fat, or fat meat, or butter; or be mashed after they are cooked, or eaten with oil or butter.

If there be an exception to this general rule—which may seem to be rather sweeping—it should be in favor of a little sweet oil on rice, or on bread puddings. But the common practice, founded upon the apparent belief that we can scarcely eat anything until it is well covered with lard or butter, is quite objectionable—nay, it is even disgusting. No pure stomach would ever prefer oily bread, or pudding, or beans, or peas; and most people would abhor the sight of such a strange combination, were not habit, in its power to change our very nature, almost omnipotent.

### SEC. 10. *Remarks on Fruit.*

There is a very great diversity of opinion on the subject of fruit. Some maintain that all fruit, even in the most ripe and perfect state, is of doubtful utility, especially for children. Others say none is hurtful, if ripe, and eaten in moderate quantity. Some require care in making a proper selection; but here again, in regard to what constitutes a proper selection, there is a difference of opinion. Some consider fruits easy of digestion; others believe they are digested only with very great difficulty.

When the cholera prevailed in the large cities of the United States, a majority of the physicians believed all fruits, even those which were ripe, to be injurious in their tendency. But it was insisted by the minority—I think very justly—that whenever fruit appeared to be injurious, it was accidental—that is, the disease, being prepared to make its attack just at that time, happened to do so immediately after the use of fruit, rather than something else, and especially in the *season* of fruits—or on account of excess; or (which was certainly the case in some instances) because the quality of the fruit was bad.

At present, the *weight* of testimony on this subject—estimating according to talent, and not according to numbers—is in favor of good fruit, used with moderation—even in the face of the cholera. Dr. Dunglison—one of the last to adopt such an opinion—appears to be in its favor.

On several points, in regard to fruit, I believe that among medical men there is no essential difference of opinion. As I always prefer, in controversies, to see in how many things antagonists agree, before proceeding to the points in which they differ, I will here endeavor to enumerate them.

1. All unripe fruits, especially, if eaten raw and uncooked—let the season, or prevalent disease, or individual, be what or who it may—are

unwholesome.

2. Excess, in the use of the most wholesome fruits, under any circumstances, is also injurious.

3. Fruits, eaten immediately after a full meal, when the stomach is in an improper condition for receiving anything more, contribute to overtask the digestive powers, and must hence produce more or less of injury.

4. The skins and kernels of the larger fruits are unwholesome, because indigestible. The skins of fruits, if beaten or masticated finely; may appear to be digested, because dissolved; but I have already endeavored to show that solution is not always digestion.

5. Fruits of all kinds are most wholesome in their own country, and in their own appropriate season.

6. Dried fruits are less wholesome than fresh.

7. Fruit of all kinds should be withheld from infants, until they have teeth.

Thus far, as I have already said, all agree; at least so far as I know. There are several other points on which medical men are generally agreed, though not universally. One of these is, that fruits, if eaten at all, should usually form a part of a regular meal. Another is, that it is better not to eat them immediately before going to bed.

There are contradictory opinions among the mass of the community, physicians as well as others, on the general intention of our summer fruits. From the fact that children's diseases prevail more at the season of the year when fruits are more abundant, many think the fruits are the immediate cause of them. Others, and with better reason, suppose that the latter are intended by the Author of nature to check or prevent the bowel diseases of summer.

Nothing, certainly, is more unnatural than to suppose that at the very season of the year when so many other influences combine to awaken a tendency to disease in the human system, the Creator should place before our eyes an abundance of fruits, inviting us by all their cooling and tempting properties, only to do us mischief. On the contrary, it seems to me much more probable that many of them were designed for our moderate use. In what quantity, under what circumstances, and which are best, it is left to human experience to determine.

Some say that fruit should never be eaten in the morning, before breakfast. Now everything I know of the human constitution, together with what I have learned from experience and observation, has been for years leading me to the contrary opinion. Indeed, I am most fully convinced, that of all periods for eating fruit, whether we use it alone or make it a part of our regular meals, the morning, soon after we rise, is the most favorable. [Footnote: I ought to remark, that as the morning is the best time for eating *good* fruit, so it is the very worst time for eating it if *not* good; and as a large proportion of that which is eaten is unripe, or otherwise bad, this may account for the general prejudice against eating it at this period.] My reasons are as follows:

1. The rest and sleep of the preceding night has restored our general vigor, and consequently has invigorated the stomach, so that digestion will be more easily and perfectly accomplished.

2. We have been, at our rising, so long without food on our stomachs, that they are not likely to be oppressed by a moderate quantity of good, ripe, wholesome fruit. In the course of our waking hours, meals follow each other in such quick succession, and there is so much variety, even at the plainest tables, to tempt us to excess, that there is more danger of injury from the addition of fruit than at our first rising.

3. I have never known any one to receive injury from the use of fruit in this way, provided no other circumstance in relation to quantity, quality, &c. had been disregarded. In my own case, the practice has, on the contrary, seemed beneficial.

4. There is one reason in favor of this practice which perhaps would have less weight, if people rose as early in the morning as they ought; or, in the language of Dr. Franklin to the inhabitants of Paris, if they knew that the sun gives light as soon as he rises. I allude to the demand which I conceive that the stomach makes for something, after so long fasting, and the pernicious custom of late breakfasts. I am persuaded that it is advisable to

eat something nearly as soon as we rise, be it never so early; and if we can get nothing else for breakfast, and have not accustomed ourselves to relish a piece of good bread, or some other simple thing, which requires no labor of preparation, I think it perfectly proper to eat a small quantity of fruit.

We come now to the particular consideration of some of those fruits which universal experience has shown to be the most salutary.

Of all these, none is more wholesome than the apple. There is indeed a great diversity in the quality even of this single article. Sweet apples are the most nutritious; but perhaps those which are gently acid, and at the same time mealy, are rather more cooling, and when eaten raw, and in the heat of summer, not less wholesome.

Apples which come to maturity very early in the season appear, as a general rule, to be less rich, and even less perfect, than those which ripen later. In view of this fact, some writers have endeavored to dissuade us from their use; and among others, Mr. Locke. We may judge a little what his opinions were, from his concluding remarks on the subject:—"I never knew apples hurt anybody," says he, "after October."

But although neither apples nor any other fruits which ripen uncommonly early are quite so good as those which come in a little later, yet I do not think they are to be wholly rejected, unless they have been raised in hot houses. Fruits, and indeed vegetables in general, whose maturity is hastened by artificial processes, must be less wholesome than when brought to perfection in nature's own appropriate time and manner. I ought to say, however, very distinctly, that of the fruits of any particular tree, those which first ripen are always the worst; for they are usually wormy, or otherwise defective.

Most of the fruit, as well as other vegetables, brought to our city markets in this country, is utterly unfit to be eaten. Sometimes it is immature; sometimes it has a hot house maturity; sometimes it has been picked so long that it has begun to decay. Many fruits—berries especially—are in perfection for a very short period only. Mulberries, for example—one kind especially—are not in perfection long enough to carry to the market house, even though the distance were very small. Luckily, however, very few mulberries are eaten. But the raspberry and strawberry, if perfect when gathered, have usually begun to decay, before they are purchased. That this appears to be rather unfrequent, is because they are gathered before they are ripe.

Dr. Dewees regards most fruits as difficult of digestion. I do not think they are so, if perfect and ripe. The experiments of Dr. Beaumont, so far as they prove any general principle, show conclusively that mellow sweet apples are more quickly digested than any kind of vegetable food whatever, except rice and sago. But even admitting they were slow of digestion, I do not think—as I have already shown in another place—that they ought on that account to be excluded. Besides, my opinion differs from that of Dr. D. in regard to the strength of the digestive powers of children. After teething, they seem to me to be able to digest any substances which adults can; and with as little difficulty.

But to return:—No fruit is in perfection longer than the apple. Besides, no fruit appears to be less injured in its nature and properties by picking it a little before it is ripe, and preserving it during the winter. It is on this account, more perhaps than any other, that I value it more highly than all other fruits united.

Apples may be used either raw or cooked. In either case, the skins and seeds should be avoided, as has been before suggested. I am not ignorant that WILLICH, in his "Lectures on Diet and Regimen"—an excellent work, in the main—says that the seeds ought to be eaten; but I believe few physiologists would comply with his injunction, especially when it is considered that he recommends, in the same connection, that we swallow the stones of cherries and plums. Strange how far our theories will sometimes carry us!

The apple is excellent when roasted or baked, especially the sweet apple. It is very common, in some places, to eat baked sweet apples with milk; and the practice is by no means a bad one. Indeed, baked or raw apples might be advantageously made a part of at least one of our meals every day. There is said to be a miserly farmer—a single gentleman—in the western part of the state of Massachusetts, who has lived on nothing but apples for his food, and water for his drink, about forty years. And yet he is said to enjoy the most perfect health. I do not propose this as an example worthy of imitation; but it shows that apples maybe made to subserve an important purpose in diet. And though I have more than once expressed an opinion highly unfavorable to the exclusive use of any one article of diet  yet if I were to confine myself to any one thing, I know of nothing except bread that I should prefer to good apples. Still, however, I prefer a variety—sweet, sour, early, late, &c.; and I should use them raw, roasted, baked, made into sauce with new or unfermented cider, and boiled. Good apples, eaten raw, with bread, form not only a very wholesome, but, to an unperverted appetite, a most delicious dinner.

Much has been said about cutting down orchards; but the whole seems to me idle—for if the fruit is of a good quality, it may be used as food, either for man or beast. And if not good, the trees ought either to be destroyed or replaced by those that will produce fruit which is better—even if the object were to make it into cider. I have said that apples may be used both by man and beast. It is well known that most domestic animals thrive well on good apples, especially sweet ones. Very tolerable molasses is also sometimes made from sweet apples.

Nearly everything which has been said above in regard to apples, will apply to pears. The best varieties of this excellent fruit are quite as nutritious and as wholesome as the apple; and as much improved for the table by baking. I believe, however, that no cheap process has yet been devised for keeping them as long in the winter. They may be preserved in the form of sauce, prepared in the same way with common apple sauce. The skins, of many kinds of pears are less injurious than those of apples; but even the skins of pears need not be eaten.

Some kinds of peaches are tolerably wholesome; but the stringy character of their pulp appears to me to render them less so than apples and pears, though I am not confident on this point. But if used at all, they should be used in less quantity at one time. Tempting as their flavor is, I seldom eat them, when I can get apples and pears; holding myself in duty bound to use the *best*, even of the fruits.

"Fruit," says Mr. Locke, "makes one of the most difficult chapters in the government of health, especially that of children. Our first parents ventured Paradise for it; and it is no wonder our children cannot stand the temptation, though it cost them their health. The regulation of this cannot come under any one general rule; for I am by no means of their mind who would keep children wholly from fruit, as a thing totally unwholesome for them, by which strict way they make them but the more ravenous after it, to eat good or bad, ripe or unripe, all that they can get, whenever they come at it.

"Melons, peaches, most sorts of plums, and all sorts of grapes, in *England*, I think children should be wholly kept from, as having a very tempting taste, in a very unwholesome juice, so that if it were possible, they should never so much as see them, or know that there was any such thing. But strawberries, cherries, gooseberries and currants, when thoroughly ripe, I think may be pretty safely allowed them."

Excellent as these remarks are, in general, I do not like his entire interdiction of the use of melons, peaches, plums, and grapes, even in England. Peaches, to be sure, as they come at a season when apples or pears, or both of them—which are more wholesome than peaches—are abundant, may be better omitted, delicious as they are to the taste; and I do not think very highly of plums. But melons, in very moderate quantity, and grapes, if we eat nothing but the ripe pulp, rejecting both the husk and the interior hard part, including the seeds, are, I think, useful and wholesome. On the other hand, I should never place cherries and gooseberries in the same list with strawberries; for the latter are, if I may use the expression, infinitely the most wholesome.

Many seem to think that not to eat all sorts of fruits is to despise, or at least to treat with neglect the gifts of God, intended for our reception; by which they mean, if they mean anything, that the use of all sorts of fruits is already found out, even in the present comparative infancy of the world. Now I do not suppose that God has made anything in vain—absolutely so—though I do not think we have found out the true uses of half the things which he has made and given us. And among those things of which we are yet ignorant, are some of the fruits. I do not believe it follows, necessarily, that because fruits are created, we are obliged to use them all.

Besides, if this is a rule, it is one which nobody follows. Every one uses more of some sorts, and fewer of others; and a large proportion of the community entirely reject some kinds. Now if the statement commonly made, that all fruits are the gifts of God, and ought therefore to be used by all persons, is correct, those who make the statement ought to conform to it as a rule of their lives, and to eat all kinds of fruit which the season and country affords; and not only eat all kinds, but see that the whole of every kind is consumed; since to waste any portion is to slight the good gifts of God.

The result then is, that we cannot obey such a rule; but are driven back to the mode which common sense dictates, which is, to make a selection, using some, and rejecting others. And the value of studying the nature of these fruits, by examining the experience of mankind in regard to them, consists in the aid thus afforded us in making our selection wisely.

There is one very common error in the use of the smaller summer fruits, such as strawberries, whortleberries, currants, &c., which is that of mixing cream, wine, spices, sugar, &c., with them. We are thus tempted to eat too great a quantity at once. Besides—which is a worse evil—we change the proportions of the saccharine parts, and thus do all in our power, by increasing a similarity in all fruits, to destroy that agreeable variety which God has established, and which is probably salutary.

## SEC. 11. *Confectionary.*

By confectionary we here mean the substances usually sold at those shops in our cities distinguished by the general name of confectionaries, and which consist either wholly of sugar, or of sugar and some other substances combined.

As to the use of a moderate quantity of pure sugar at our meals, whether it is procured at a confectioner's shop or elsewhere, I do not know that there is any strong objection to it; though I believe that it cannot be regarded as indispensable to health—for were that the fact, it seems to me to imply something short of infinite wisdom in the creation of articles destined for our sustenance. But I have spoken on this subject elsewhere.

A part, however, of the contents of the confectionary shop are actually poisonous. I refer to those things which are either frosted, as it is called, or colored. The substances applied to the sugar for this purpose are usually some mineral or vegetable poison; although the fact of its being a poison may not always be known to the manufacturer. The most unhappy consequences have occasionally followed the use of confectionary, when poisoned in this manner. A family of four persons, in New York, were made sick in this way in March of year before last, and some of them came very near losing their lives. The "frosting" which caused the mischief was pronounced by eminent chemists to be one fifth rank poison.[Footnote: It is to be remembered that those who eat confectionary so slightly poisoned that it does not make them sick at once, may nevertheless be as much injured in their constitutions as they who are poisoned outright. In the latter case, the poison is in part thrown out of the body; in the former, it remains in it much longer—and therefore more surely, though more slowly, accomplishes the work of destruction.] The coloring substances used are sometimes poisonous, as well as the frosting.

Some of the articles sold at these shops consist of sugar mixed with paste. Others are called sweetmeats; that is, fruits, or rinds of fruits, preserved in sugar. All these substances, I believe, without exception, are injurious.

The great evils of confectionary yet remain to be mentioned. These are of three kinds, physical, mental and moral.

Some of the *physical* evils have, it is true, just been mentioned; but there is another evil of still greater magnitude. Young people who eat confectionary, commonly eat it between meals. This produces mischief in two ways. First, it keeps the stomach at work when it ought to rest; for this, like every other muscular organ, requires its seasons of repose. Secondly, it destroys gradually the appetite; so that when the regular meal arrives, the accustomed keenness of appetite does not come with it. And the consequence is, not so much that we do not eat enough, as that we are fastidious, and eat a little of this, then a little of that; and usually select the worst things. We are not hungry enough to make a meal of a single article of plain food. And this evil goes on increasing, as long as we have access to the confectionary shop. These statements describe the case of thousands of pupils, of both sexes, at our schools and seminaries.

The *intellectual* evil resulting from the use of confectionary consists in the fondness for excitement which is produced. You will seldom find a person who depends daily and almost hourly on some excitement to his appetite and stomach, and is not satisfied with plain food, who will content himself to *study* without unnatural excitements of the mind. Duty to himself or to others will not move him. He must have before him the hope of reward, or the fear of punishment. He must be moved by emulation or ambition, or some other questionable or wicked motive or passion.

But the *moral* results, to the young, of using confectionary, are still more dreadful. I do not here refer to the danger of meeting with bad company at the shops themselves, or of going from these places of pollution *directly* to the grog-shop, the gambling-house, or the brothel; though there is danger enough, even here. But I allude to the tendency which a habit of not resting satisfied with plain food, but of depending on exciting things, has, to make us dissatisfied with plain moral enjoyments—the society of friends, and the quiet discharge of our duty to God and our neighbor. Just in proportion as we gratify our propensity for excitement at the confectioner's shop, just in the same proportion do we expose ourselves to the, danger of yielding to temptation, should other gratifications present themselves. The young of both sexes who are in the use of confectionary, are on the high road to gluttony, drunkenness, or debauchery; perhaps to all three. I do not say they will certainly arrive there, for circumstances not quite miraculous may pluck them as "brands from the burning;" but I do not hesitate to say that such is the inevitable tendency; and I call on every mother and teacher who reads this section, to beware of confectionaries, and see, if possible, that the young never set foot in them. They are a road through which thousands pass to the chamber of death—death to the immortal spirit, as well as to the body, its vehicle.

More might be added—for this is an important subject—but I trust I have said enough. Those who have read and believe what I have written, if they remain wholly unaffected and unmoved, would not be roused to effort were anything to be added.

## SEC. 12. *Pastry.*

Dr. Paris, a distinguished British writer on diet, says that all pastry is "an abomination." And yet, go where we will, we find it often on the table. Hardly any one, whether old or young, attempts to do without it.

There are indeed some, who will not eat pie-crust, or high-seasoned cakes formed of paste; but yet will not hesitate to eat hot bread, or rolls, or biscuits made of wheat flour, bolted. Now what is this but paste? If we could see the contents of the stomach, an hour after the mass is swallowed, we should find it to be paste, and *mere* paste.

And yet the evil is increasing everywhere. So generally is this true, that a person who refuses to eat hot bread, or cake, or biscuit, is deemed singular. He who ventures to lift his voice against it is deemed an ascetic or a visionary. But such a voice must be raised, and heard, too, whether its monitions are or are not regarded.

Pastry is less objectionable, however, when used in the form of hot bread, &c., than when butter or fat is mixed with it. Then it becomes one of the most indigestible substances in the world. Besides, it not only tries the patience of the stomach, but according to Willich, whose authority ranks high, it tends to produce diseases of the skin, especially a disease which he calls "copper in the face," and which he pronounces incurable.

I know not whether the eruptions so common on the faces of young people in this country, and especially of young men, are in every instance either produced or aggravated by pastry; but I am very sure of one thing, viz., that those who are in the use of pastry, and have eruptions of the skin of any kind, will not be apt to get well, as long as they continue the use of this objectionable substance.

Physicians are often consulted about eruptions on the face. When they assign the real cause, which is undoubtedly connected with the improper gratification of some of the appetites, in one way or another, it is seldom that the patient has self-command enough to follow his prescription of temperance or abstinence. Mothers, it is yours to prevent this mischief;—first, by establishing correct physical habits; secondly, by teaching your children the great duty of self-denial—not only by precept, but by your own good example.

## SEC. 13. *Crude or Raw Substances.*

I have reserved this section for remarks on certain articles used at our fashionable modern tables, of which I could not well find it convenient to speak elsewhere. And first, of SALADS, and HERBS used in cooking; such as asparagus, artichokes, spinage, plantain, cabbage, dock, lettuce, water-cresses, chives, &c.

Several of these substances are often eaten raw, in which state they are exceedingly indigestible, at the best; and they are rendered still more beyond the reach of the powers of the stomach, by the oil or vinegar which is added to them. Boiled, they are more tolerable; especially asparagus. In the midst, however, of such an abundance of excellent food as this country affords, it is most surprising that anybody should ever take it into their heads to eat such crude substances; and above all, that they should fill children's stomachs with them. What child, with an unperverted appetite, would not prefer a good ripe apple, or peach, or pear, to the most approved raw salads?—and a good baked one, to the best boiled asparagus?

NUTS, in general, are probably made for other animals rather than man; though of this we cannot in the present infancy of human knowledge be quite certain. But if any of them were intended, by the Creator, for man, it is the chesnut; and this should be boiled. Boiled chesnuts are used as food, in many parts of southern Europe; and to a very considerable extent.

SPICES, as they are sometimes called, such as nutmeg, mace, pepper, pimento; cubebs, cardamoms, juniper berries, ginger, calamus, cloves, cinnamon, caraway, coriander, fennel, parsley, dill, sage, marjoram, thyme, pennyroyal, lavender, hyssop, peppermint, &c., are unfit for the human stomach—above all in infancy—except as medicines.

There are several other vegetables equally objectionable with the last, though they cannot be classed under the same head. Such are mustard, horseradish, raw onions, garlic, cucumbers, and pickles. No appetite which has not been accustomed to these substances in early infancy, will ever require them. Not that they may not sometimes be useful in enabling the stomach—at every age—to get rid of certain substances with which it has been improperly or unreasonably loaded;—this is undoubtedly the fact; ardent spirits would do the same. And it is with a view to some such effect, generally, that medical writers have spoken in their favor. Some of them stimulate the stomach to get rid of a load of *green* fruit; others, of a load of *fat* or *salt* food; others, again, of too large a *quantity* of food which is naturally wholesome.

But in all these cases, they should be considered, not as food, but as medicine; and we ought to call them by their right name. And if we withhold the cause of the disease, there will be no need of the medicine.

# CHAPTER VIII.

## DRINKS.

Infants need little drink. Adults, even, generally drink to cool themselves. Simple water the best drink. Opinions of Dr. Oliver and Dr. Dewees. Animal food increases thirst. Only one real drink in the world. The true object of all drink. Tea, coffee, chocolate, beer, &c. Milk and water, molasses and water, &c. Cider, wine, and ardent spirits. Bad food and drink the most prolific sources of disease. Children naturally prefer water. Danger of hot drinks. Cold drinks. Mischief they produce. Caution to mothers. Extracts. Drinking cold water, while hot.

Children need little if any drink, so long as their food is nothing but milk; nor indeed for some time afterward, unless they are indulged in the use of animal food. Adults, even, very seldom drink merely to quench natural thirst. In the summer, people usually drink either to cool themselves, or to gratify a thirst which is wholly artificial. Tea, coffee, beer, cider, and most other common drinks, when not used for the sake of their coolness, are drank, both in winter and summer, for this purpose.

That this is the fact, we have the most abundant and unequivocal evidence. I know that much is said of the demand which a profuse perspiration creates among hard laborers in the summer. Such a sudden abstraction of a large amount of fluid requires, it is said, a proportional supply, or life would soon become extinct. Yet there are many old men who have perspired profusely at their labor all their days, and yet have drank nothing at all, except their tea, morning and evening; and perhaps have eaten, for one or two of their meals daily, in summer, a bowl of bread and milk. And some of them are among the most remarkable instances of longevity which the country affords.

How the system acquires a sufficient supply of moisture to keep up good health, in these cases, I do not pretend to determine: perhaps it is through the medium of the lungs. But at any rate, it can obtain it without our drinking for that sole purpose, to the great danger of exciting liver complaints, diarrhoea, dyspepsia, colds, rheumatisms, and fevers.

But if adults who perspire freely do not require much drink, children certainly do not; and above all, young children. And if they do require any thing, it is only simple water. The following remarks of Dr. Oliver, of Hanover, N.H., are extracted from Dr. Mussey's late Prize Essay on Ardent Spirits:

> "Who has not observed the extreme satisfaction which children derive from quenching their thirst with pure water? And who that has perverted his appetite for drink, by stimulating his palate with bitter beer, sour cider, rum and water, and other beverages of human invention, but would be a gainer, even on the score of mere animal gratification, without any reference to health, if he could bring back his vitiated taste to the simple relish of nature?
>
> "Children drink because they are dry. Grown people drink, whether dry or not, because they have discovered a way of making drink pleasant. Children drink water because this is a beverage of nature's own brewing, which she has made for the purpose of quenching a natural thirst. Grown people drink anything but water, because this fluid is intended to quench only a natural thirst; and natural thirst is a thing which they seldom feel."

There is a great deal of truth, as well as of sound philosophy, in these two paragraphs, and little less of truth in the following paragraph from Dr. Dewees:

> "We have witnessed very often, with sorrow, parents giving to their young children wine, or other stimulating liquors. Nature never intended anything stronger than water to be the drink for children. This they enjoy greatly; and much advantage is occasionally experienced from its use, especially after they have commenced the use of animal food."

Two things are to be observed in the last remarks, which are, that children demand drink of any kind but seldom, and that even this occasional demand is often the special result of the use of animal food. Here comes out an important secret. It is the use of animal food, to a very great degree, in adults and children both, that creates so much of that unnatural thirst which prevails in the community. When we shall come to lay aside animal food, in childhood, youth, manhood and age, much that is now *called* thirst will be banished; and much of the intemperance and other kinds of sensuality which follow in its train.

It has been sometimes said that there is but one kind of drink in the world —and that is water. This is strictly, or rather *physiologically* true. For, though many mixtures are *called* drinks, it is only the water which they contain that answers any of the legitimate purposes for which drink was intended by the Creator.

The object of drink, besides quenching our thirst, or rather *while* it quenches it, is, not to be digested, like food, but to pass directly from the stomach into the blood-vessels, and dilute and temper the blood, rendering it more fit to answer the great purpose of sustaining life and health. Now, there is nothing that can do this but water. Alcohol cannot do it, nor can turpentine, oil, quicksilver, melted lead, or any other liquid.

Tea, coffee, chocolate, small beer, soda water, lemonade, &c., which are nearly all water, quench the thirst very well, it is true; but not quite so well as water alone would. The narcotic principle of the first two, the alcoholic principle of the fourth, and the mucilage, nutriment, acid, and alkali of the rest, are in the way; for thirst would be quenched still better without them, even when it is of an unnatural kind.

Indeed, the same or similar remarks may be made in regard to all other mixtures which are usually proposed as drinks. Even milk and water, molasses and water, &c., in favor of which so much is said, are objectionable, as mere drinks. Not that they contain anything poisonous, but they evidently contain nutriment; and even this, except as a part or the whole of a regular meal, does harm; for it sets the stomach at work when it needs repose. Mere drink, as I have already said, is never digested.

But if the drinks above mentioned, and even milk and water, are objectionable, what shall we say of cider, wine, and ardent spirits?—substances which contain, the latter one half, and the two former from one twentieth to one fourth alcohol. Surely, nobody will deny that these substances ought, at all events, to be banished from the nursery. And yet we occasionally find them there, not only for the use of the mother, to the ruin of the child, indirectly—but also, in some of their smoother forms, for the use of the child itself.

I would not lay too much stress on food and drink; for, as I have already observed, more than once, the causes of infantile ill health and mortality are numerous. Still I must insist that, of all the sources of disease, these are the most prolific. Much is done towards ruining the health of children by the improper food and drink of the mother. But when, in addition to all this, the children themselves are early fed with animal food, and with stimulating drinks—punch, coffee, tea, &c.—and an artificial thirst is early excited and rendered habitual, their destruction, for time and eternity, is almost inevitable.

Very few children relish any drink but water, or sweetened water, at first; and where they do, it is probably hereditary. I have been struck with their tastes and preferences; nor less with the folly of those around them, in endeavoring to change them, by requiring them—almost always against their will—to sip a little coffee, or a little tea, or a little lemonade; or, it may be, a little toddy. Such children *may* escape the death of the drunkard or the debauchee; but if they do, it will not be through the instrumentality of the parents.

I am very much opposed to giving children hot drinks of any kind. If they are to drink substances which are injurious, as tea or coffee, let them be cool. I do not say *cold*, for that would be going to the other extreme. But no drink, in any ordinary case, should be above the heat of our bodies; that is, about 98 degrees of Fahrenheit's thermometer. Yet the precautions of this paragraph will be almost unnecessary, if children are confined—as they ought to be, and would be, did we not go out of our way to teach them otherwise—to water, as their only drink. Cold water is almost always preferred. Not one child in a thousand would ever prefer it hot, until his taste had been perverted. No writer has inveighed more against hot drinks of every kind, than the late William Cobbett—and, as I think, with more justice.

But, in avoiding one rock, we must not, as has already been intimated, make shipwreck on another. Hot drinks, though they injure the powers of the stomach, and by that means and through that medium, are one principal cause of the almost universal early decay of teeth, are yet less injurious, or at least less dangerous, immediately, than cold ones. Mr. Locke, in speaking of the sports of a child, in the open air, has the following quaint, but judicious remarks:

"Playing in the open air has but this one danger in it, that I know; and that is, that when he is hot with running up and down, he should sit or lie down on the cold or moist earth. This, I grant, and drinking cold drink, when they are hot with labor or exercise, brings more people to the grave, or to the brink of it, by fevers and other diseases, than anything I know. These mischiefs are easily enough prevented when he is little, being then seldom out of sight. And if, during his childhood, he be constantly and rigorously kept from sitting on the ground, or drinking any cold liquor, while he is hot, the custom of forbearing, grown into *habit*, will help much to preserve him, when he is no longer under his maid's or tutor's eye.

"More fevers and surfeits are got by people's drinking when they are hot, than by any one thing I know. If he (the child) be very hot, he should by no means *drink*; at least a good piece of bread, first to be eaten, will gain time to warm his drink *blood hot*, which then he may drink safely. If he be very dry, it will go down so warmed, and quench his thirst better; and if he will not drink it so warmed, abstaining will not hurt him. Besides, this will teach him to forbear, which is a habit of the greatest use for health of mind and body too."

The last remarks are full of wisdom. Mothers may depend upon it, that every indulgence to which they accustom their children paves the way for *habitual* indulgence; and has a tendency to lead, indirectly, to indulgence in other matters; and, on the contrary, every self-denial which they can lead children to exercise, voluntarily—even in these every-day matters of food, drink, exercise, &c. is so much gained in the great work of self-denial and the resisting of temptation in matters of higher importance. But I must not moralize too long; having dwelt on this same point under the head Confectionary. I proceed, therefore, to make a few more extracts from Mr. Locke:

"Not being permitted to *drink* without eating, will prevent the custom of having the cup often at his nose; a dangerous beginning."

"Men often bring habitual hunger and thirst on themselves by custom."

"You may, if you please, bring any one to be thirsty every hour."

"I once lived in a house, where, to appease a froward child, they gave him *drink* as often as he cried, so that he was constantly bibbing. And though he could not speak, yet he drank more in twenty-four hours than I did."

"It is convenient, for health and sobriety, to drink no more than natural thirst requires; and he that eats not salt meats, nor drinks strong drink, will seldom thirst between meals."

Great mischief is often done to their health by children at school; and one instance of this is, in getting violently heated with exercise, and then pouring down large quantities of cold water to cool themselves. I once made it a habitual rule for pupils, that they must drink water, if they drank it at all, on leaving their seats to go to their plays, but not afterwards: and I was so situated that I could prevent the law from being broken, as there was no spring or well to which they could have access, privately. And though they thought the rule rather severe, I have no doubt it saved them from much injury, and perhaps sometimes from sickness.

# CHAPTER IX.

## GIVING MEDICINE.

"Prevention" better than "cure." Nine in ten infantile diseases caused by errors in diet and drink. Signs of failing health. Causes of a bad breath. Flesh eaters. Gormandizers. General rule for preventing disease. When to call a physician.

So much error prevails in regard to the medical management of the young, that a volume might be written without exhausting the subject. [Footnote: Such a volume is in preparation. It is intended as a companion to the present.] My present limits and plan allow of only a few remarks, and those must be general.

That "an ounce of prevention is worth a pound of cure," has so long ago become a proverb, that it seems almost idle to repeat the sentiment. And yet it is to be feared that very few receive it as a practical truth, in the management of children. Now nothing is more certain than that it is easier, as well as more humane, to prevent diseases than to cure them.

I have elsewhere mentioned the opinion of a very eminent physician, that nine in ten of children's diseases may be imputed to error with regard to the quantity or the quality of their food. For myself, I am by no means certain that nine out of ten is the exact proportion, though I think the number is, at all events, very large. Few children, or even grown persons, are seized with disease suddenly. Their progress towards it is always gradual, and sometimes imperceptible. To a physician of any tolerable degree of skill, however, there is no difficulty in observing and pointing out the first steps towards illness; in those whose habits of life are well known to him; and of foretelling the consequence.

But since parents and nurses are not so well qualified as physicians to make these observations, I will endeavor to point out a few certain signs and symptoms by which they may know a child's health to be declining, even before be appears to be sick.—For if these are neglected, the evil increases, goes on from bad to worse, and more violent and apparent complaints will follow, and perhaps end in incurable diseases, which a timely remedy, or a slight change in the diet and manner of life, would have infallibly prevented.

"The first tendency to disease," says Dr. Cadogan, "may be observed in a child's breath. It is not enough that the breath is not offensive; it should be sweet and fragrant, like a nosegay of fresh flowers, or a pail of new milk from a young cow that feeds upon the sweetest grass of the spring; and this as well at first waking in the morning, as all day long." [Footnote: Buchan's "Advice to Mothers," pages 337, 388]

There is much of truth in these remarks; but if they are wholly true, then very few children are perfectly healthy. For no child that eats much animal food of any sort, or, what amounts to nearly the same thing, much butter or gravy, will long retain the fragrant breath here alluded to. Who has not observed the difference in this respect, between animals in general which feed on flesh, and those which feed on grass? And whether it is the character of their respective food that makes the difference or not, it is also true that there is nearly as much difference of breath between *men* who use animal food and those who do not, as between other animals. The breath of some of our enormous meat eaters would almost remind one of a slaughter house.

Nor is it the quality of food alone, that will induce a foul breath, either in adults or infants. He who swallows such enormous quantities, even of plain food, as by overloading and fatiguing the stomach, tend gradually to debilitate it, will produce the same effect. The enormous feeders of this full feeding country, whether they are young or old, whether they inhabit the mountain or the vale, and whether they feed on animal food or not, have generally a bad breath; and if they seldom offend, it is because few feed otherwise. And it is not too much—in my own opinion—to say of this whole class of gormandizers, no less than of the flesh eaters, that they have laid for themselves the foundation of future disease.

One general rule may here be distinctly laid down. As a child's breath becomes hot and feverish, or strong, or acid, we may be certain that "digestion and surfeit have fouled and disturbed the blood; and now is the time to apply a proper remedy, and prevent a train of impending evils. Let the child be restrained in its food. Let it eat less, live upon milk or thin broth for a day or two, and be carried (or walk if it is able) a little more than usual in the open air." [Footnote: Advice to Mothers, page 338]

This rule is the more important, because, if duly persevered in, it will generally prevent disease, and save the trouble and evil consequences of taking medicine at all. Meanwhile it will be advisable to call in a physician—not to give drugs, but to prevent the necessity of giving them. There is a foolish fear abroad that physicians, if called before a person is violently sick, will dose him with their drugs, as a matter of course, till they *make* him sick. But this, no judicious physician will ever do. It may *have been* done, though I believe it has been seldom. The more general course is to defer calling for medical advice, till it is too late to use preventive means; and medicine is then resorted to by the physician as a sort of necessary evil.

A judicious physician, seasonably called in, would in many instances save a severe fit of sickness, besides a great deal of expense, both of time and money.

But if the first symptoms of approaching disease are overlooked—if the child is fed, or rather crammed; with solid food as much as ever—and if no medical advice is sought, his sleep will soon become disturbed; he will be talking, starting, and tumbling about, and will have frightful dreams; or he will at other times be found smiling and laughing. To these, in the end, may be added, loss of appetite, paleness, emaciation, weakness, cough, and consumption; or colics, worms, and convulsions.

I do not undertake to say that the most judicious parental management, aided by the greatest medical skill, will always prevent disease; far from it. The child may and undoubtedly sometimes does inherit a tendency to a particular disease; or he may be made sick by error in regard to dress, exercise, &c. But so long as nine tenths of the disease and early mortality of the young might be prevented by due attention to all these means combined, so long will it be necessary to reiterate the sentiments of the present section.

# CHAPTER X.

## EXERCISE.

SEC. 1. Objections to the use of cradles.—SEC. 2. Carrying in the arms—its uses and abuses.—SEC. 3. Creeping—why useful—to be encouraged.—SEC. 4. Walking—general directions about it.—SEC. 5. Riding abroad in carriages.—SEC. 6. Riding on horseback—objections. Riding schools.

This subject may be considered under the following heads: ROCKING IN THE CRADLE; CARRYING IN THE ARMS; CREEPING; WALKING; RIDING IN A CARRIAGE; AND RIDING ON HORSEBACK. These I shall consider in their order.

### SEC. 1. *Rocking in the Cradle.*

There are two opinions in regard to the use of the cradle in the nursery. Some condemn it altogether; others think its occasional use highly proper. Those who condemn it, do it chiefly on the ground that it produces a whirling motion of the brain, which, while it inclines to giddiness and lulls to sleep, disturbs, in some degree, the process of digestion.

It seems to me that there is weight to this objection; and although the cradle has been extensively used without producing any obviously evil effects, I should greatly prefer to have it universally laid aside. As far as mere amusement is demanded, it is quite unnecessary, since there are so many amusements which are far better. As a means of inducing sleep, I am still more strongly opposed to it; for if a child be rationally treated in every other respect, it will never need artificial means to induce it to sleep. Nature will then be the most appropriate directress in this matter.

If there is a cradle in a nursery, it is almost always full of clothes loaded with air more or less impure, and the child is buried in it more than is compatible with health, even in the judgment of the mother or the nurse; for so convenient is its use, and so great the temptation to keep the child in it, that he will often be found soaking there a large proportion of his time. Every one knows that the air has not so free access to a child in the cradle as elsewhere, especially if it have a kind of covering or hood to it, as we often see. Besides, the cradle is a piece of furniture which takes up a great deal of space in the nursery; and every one who has made the trial effectually, will, it seems to me, greatly prefer its room to its company.

If any cradle is to be used, those are best which are suspended by cords, and are swung, rather than rocked. And this swinging should be in a line with the body of the child as much as possible; as this motion is less likely to produce injury than its opposite.

## SEC. 2. *Carrying in the Arms.*

This is the most appropriate exercise for the first two months of existence; and indeed, one of the best for some time afterward.

Although a healthy, thriving child ought to sleep, for some time after birth, from two thirds to three fourths of his time, yet it should never be forgotten that the demand for proper exercise during the rest of the time, is not the less imperious on this account; but probably the more so.

I have already mentioned the importance of bathing, which is one form of exercise, and of gentle motion in the arms, immediately afterward. The same gentle motion should be often repeated during the day; care being taken to hold the child in such a position as will be easy to him, and favorable to the free exercise of all his limbs and muscles.

There are many mothers and nurses, who not only rejoice that the infant inclines to sleep a great deal, since it gives them more liberty, but who take pains to prolong these hours beyond what nature requires, by artificial means. I refer not only to the use of the cradle, but to means still more artificial—the use of cordials and opiates, to which I have already adverted. But whatever the means used may be, they defeat the purposes of nature, and are in the highest degree reprehensible. Nothing but the most chilling poverty should prevent the mother from having the child—for a few weeks of its first existence at least—in her own arms, nearly all the time which is not absolutely demanded for repose. She should even invite it to wakefulness, rather than encourage sleep.

Attention to exercise ought to be commenced before the child is more than ten days old. For this purpose he should be placed on his back, on a pillow, in order that the body may rest at as many points as possible. In this position he has the opportunity to move his limbs with the most perfect freedom, and to exercise his numerous muscles. There is nothing more important to the infant—not even sleep itself—than the action of all his muscles; and nothing contributes more to his rapid growth.

At first, the body should be kept, while on the arm, in nearly a horizontal position, with the head perhaps a very little elevated; but after a few weeks, it will be proper to change the position for a small part of the time; placing the body so that it may form an angle of a few degrees with the horizon. When this is done, however, it should always be by placing the hand against the shoulders and head, in such a manner as to support well the back; for it is extremely injurious to suffer the feeble spine to sustain, at this early period, any considerable weight.

Still more erroneous is the practice of some careless nurses, of carrying the child quite upright a part of the time, almost without any support at all. There can be no doubt that the spinal column of many a child is injured for life in this way. There can be no apology for such things.

But it is not sufficient to denounce, merely, the custom of holding the infant's body in an erect position. Every inquiring mother—and it is for such, and no other, that I write—will naturally and properly ask the reason why.

The child is not born with all its bones solid. Some are mere cartilage for a considerable time. This is the case with the bones of the back. Now every person must see that the weight of the child's head and shoulders, resting for a considerable time on the slender cartilaginous spinal column, may easily bend it. And a curvature, thus given, may, and often does, deform children for life.

Dr. Dewees mentions a nurse who, from a foolish fondness for displaying them, made the children consigned to her charge sit perfectly upright before they were a month old. It is truly ludicrous, he says, to see the little creatures sitting as straight as if they were stiffened by a back board. It is truly *horrible*, I should say, rather than ludicrous. Crooked spines must be the inevitable consequence, if nothing worse.

The practice of bracing children, as it is called, by straps, back boards, corsets, &c., where it has produced any effect at all, has always had a tendency to crook the spine. This may be seen first, by observing one shoulder to be lower than the other, and next by a projection of the part of the shoulder blades next to the spine. Whenever these changes begin to appear, it is time to send for a physician, though it may often be too late to effect a cure. But on the general subject of bracing and corseting, I have treated at sufficient length elsewhere.

There is another error committed in carrying children in the arms. The head of the infant is often permitted either to hang constantly on one side, or to roll about loosely; as if it hardly belonged to the body. In the former case there is danger of producing a habit of holding the head upon one side, which it will be very difficult to overcome; in the latter, the spinal marrow itself may be injured—which would produce alarming and perhaps fatal consequences.

But all these evils, as has already been said, may be prevented, if the hand is placed so as to support the head and shoulders. Let not the mother, however, who reads this work, trust the matter wholly to a nurse; she must see to it herself; else she incurs a most fearful responsibility. The suggestions I have made are the more important in the case of children either very fleshy or very feeble, and of those disposed to rickets or scrofula; but they are important to all.

I have said that the motion of the child, on the arm, should be gentle. Many are in the habit of tossing infants about. There can be no objection to a slight and slow movement up and down, for a minute or so at a time; indeed, it is rather to be recommended, as likely to give strength and vigor no less than pleasure to the child. But when such movements are carried to excess, so as to frighten the child, they are highly reprehensible. The shock thus produced to the nervous system has sometimes been so great as to produce sudden death. Nor is it safe to run, jump, or descend stairs hastily or violently, with a child in our arms; and for similar reasons.

Infants should not be carried always on the same arm, for there is danger of contracting a habit of leaning to one side, and thus of becoming crooked. On this account, the arm on which they rest should be often changed. Nor should they be grasped too firmly. A skilful mother will hold a child quite loosely, with the most perfect safety; while an inexperienced one will grasp him so hard as to expose the soft bones to be bent out of their place, and yet be quite as liable to let him fall as she who handles him with more ease and freedom.

### SEC. 3. *Creeping.*

"Mankind must creep before they can walk," is an old adage often used to remind us of that patient application which is so indispensable to secure any highly important or valuable end. But it is as true literally, as it is figuratively. The act of creeping exercises in a remarkable degree nearly all the muscles of the body; and this, too, without much fatigue.

Some mothers there indeed are, who think it a happy circumstance if a child can be taught to walk without this intermediate step. But such mothers must have strange ideas of the animal economy. They must never have thought of the pleasure which creeping affords the mind, or of the vigor it imparts to the body.

Children are wonderfully pleased with their own voluntary efforts. What they can do themselves, yields them ten-fold greater pleasure than if done by the mother or the nurse. Yet the latter are exceedingly prone to forget or overlook all this—and to say, at least practically, that the only proper efforts are those to which themselves give direction.

They are moreover exceedingly fond of display. Some mothers seem to act—in all they do with and for children—as if all the latter were good for, was display and amusement. They feed them, indeed, and strive to prolong their existence; but it appears to be for similar reasons to those which would lead them to take kind care of a pet lamb.

It is on this account that they dress them out in the manner they do, strive to make them sit up straight, and prohibit their creeping. It is on this account too, as much perhaps as any other, that go-carts and leading strings are put in such early requisition. The contrary would be far the safer extreme; and the parent who keeps his child scrambling about upon the back as long as possible, and when he cannot prevent longer an inversion of this position, retains him at creeping as long as is in his power, is as much wiser, in comparison with him who urges him forward to make a prodigy of him, as he is who, instead of making his child a prodigy in mind or morals at premature age, holds him back, and endeavors to have his mental and moral nature developed no faster than his physical frame.

I wish young mothers would settle it in their minds at once, that the longer their children creep the better. They need have no fears that the force of habit will retain them on their knees after nature has given them strength to rise and walk; for their incessant activity and incontrollable restlessness will be sure to rouse them as early as it ought. Least of all ought the difficulty of keeping them clean, to move them from the path of duty.

Children who are allowed to crawl, will soon be anxious to do more. We shall presently see them taking hold of a chair or a table, and endeavoring to raise themselves up by it. If they fail in a dozen attempts, they do not give up the point; but persevere till their efforts are crowned with success.

Having succeeded in raising themselves from the floor, they soon learn to stand, by holding to the object by which they have raised themselves. Soon, they acquire the art of standing without holding; [Footnote: The art of standing, which consists in balancing one's self, by means of the muscles of the body and lower limb—simple as it may seem to those who have never reflected on the subject—is really an important acquisition for a child of twelve or fifteen months. No wonder they feel a conscious pride, when they find themselves able to stand erect, like the world around them.] ere long they venture to put forward one foot—they then repeat the effort and walk a little, holding at the same time by a chair; and lastly they acquire, with joy to them inexpressible and to us inconceivable, the art of "trudging" alone.

When children learn to walk in nature's own way, it is seldom indeed that we find them with curved legs, or crooked or clubbed feet. These deformities are almost universally owing either to the mother or the nurse.

Let me be distinctly understood as utterly opposed, not only to go-carts, leading strings, and every other *mechanical* contrivance, to induce children to walk before their legs are fit for it, but to efforts of every kind, whose main object is the same. Teaching them to walk by taking hold of one of their hands, is in some respects quite as bad as any other mode; for if the child should fall while we have hold of his hand, there is some danger of dislocating or otherwise injuring the limb.

Falls we must expect; but if a child is left to his own voluntary efforts as much as possible, these falls will be fewer, and probably less serious, than under any other circumstances.

### SEC. 4. *Walking.*

"The way to learn how to write without ruled lines, is *to rule*," was the frequent saying of an old schoolmaster whom I once knew; and I may say with as much confidence and with more truth, that "the way for a child to learn to walk alone, is to hold by things."

I have anticipated, in previous pages, much of what might have otherwise been contained in this section. A few additional remarks are all that will be necessary.

At first, the nursery will be quite large enough for our young pedestrian. Much time should elapse before he is permitted to go abroad, upon the green grass;—not lest the air should reach him, or the sun shine upon his face and hands, but because the surface of the ground is so much less firm and regular than the floor, that he ought to be quite familiar with walking on the latter, in the first place.

But when he can walk well in the play ground, garden, fields, and roads, it is highly desirable that he should go out more or less every day, when the weather will possibly admit; nor would I be so fearful as many are of a drop of rain or dew, or a breath of wind. For say what they will in favor of riding, sailing, and other modes of exercise, there is none equal to walking, as soon as a child is able;—none so natural—none, in ordinary cases, so salutary. I know it is unpopular, and therefore our young master or young miss must be hoisted into a carriage, or upon the back of a horse, to the manifest danger of health or limbs, or both.

Who of us ever knew a herdsman or a shepherd who found it for the health and well-being of the young calf or lamb to hoist it into a carriage, and carry it through the streets, instead of suffering it to walk? Such a thing would excite astonishment; and the man who should do it would be deemed insane. The health and growth of our young domestic animals is best promoted by suffering them to walk, run, and skip in their own way. They ask no artificial legs, or horses, or carriages. But would it not be difficult to find arguments in favor of carrying children about, when they are able to walk, which would not be equally strong in favor of carrying about lambs and calves and pigs.

This is the more remarkable from the consideration, elsewhere urged, that in general we take more rational pains about the physical well-being of domestic animals, than of children. However, it will be seen, on a little reflection, that the number of those who carry children about, is, after all, very inconsiderable. The greater portion of the community regard it as too troublesome or costly; and if poverty brought with it no other evils than a permit to children to walk on the legs which the Creator gave them, it could hardly be deemed a misfortune.

It is scarcely necessary to add that there will be nothing gained to the young—or to persons of any age—from walks which are very long and fatiguing. Walking should refresh and invigorate: when it is carried beyond this, especially with the young child, we have passed the line of safety.

## SEC. 5. *Riding in Carriages.*

It will be seen by the foregoing section, that I am not very friendly to the use of carriages for the young, after they can walk. Before this period, however, I think they may be often serviceable; and there are occasional instances which may render them useful afterward. On this account, I have thought it might be well to give the following general directions.

Carriages for children should be so constructed as not to be liable to overset. To this end, the wheels must be low, and the axle unusually extended. The body should be long enough to allow the child to lie down when necessary; and so deep that he may not be likely to fall out. Everything should be made secure and firm, to avoid, if possible, the danger of accidents.

The carriage should be drawn steadily and slowly; not violently, or with a jerking motion. Such a place should be selected as will secure the child—if necessary—from the full blaze of a hot sun. This point might indeed be secured by having the carriage covered; but I am opposed to covered carriages, for children or adults, unless we are compelled to ride in the rain.

While the child is unable to sit up without injury, and even for some months afterwards, he ought by all means to lie down in a carriage, because it requires more strength to sit in a seat which is moving, than in a place where he is stationary. In assuming the horizontal position, in a carriage, a pillow is needed, and such other arrangements as will prevent too much rolling.

After the child's strength will fairly permit, he may sit up in the carriage, but he ought still to be secured against too much motion. As his strength increases, however, the latter direction will be less and less necessary. I need not repeat in this place, (had I not witnessed so many accidents from neglect,) the caution recently given, that great care should be taken to prevent the child from falling out of the carriage.

While children are riding abroad in cold weather, much pains should be taken to see that they are suitably clothed. It is well to keep them in motion, while they are in the carriage, and especially to guard against their falling asleep in the open air, until they have become very much accustomed to being out in it.

It has been said by some writers, that a ride ought never to exceed the length of half an hour; but no positive rule can be given, except to avoid over-fatigue.

### SEC. 6. *Riding on Horseback.*

While children are very young, I think it both improper and unsafe to take them abroad on horseback; I mean so long as they are in health. In case of disease, this mode of exercise is sometimes one of the most salutary in the world. But after boys are six or seven years old, and girls ten, if they are ever to practise horsemanship, it is time for them to begin; both because they are less apt to be unreasonably timid at this age, and because they learn much more rapidly.

So few parents are good horsemen, that if there is a riding school at hand, I should prefer placing a child in it at once. But I wish to be distinctly understood, that I do not consider it a matter of importance, especially to females, that they should ever learn to ride at all.

Some of the principal objections to riding on horseback, by boys, as an ordinary exercise, are the following:

1. Walking, as I have already intimated, is one of the most HEALTHY modes of exercise in the world. It is nature's exercise; and was unquestionably in exclusive use long before universal dominion was given to man, if not for many centuries afterward; and I believe it would be very difficult to prove that it interfered at all with human longevity; for the first of our race lived almost a thousand years.

2. Young children, in riding on horseback, are rather apt to acquire, rapidly, the habit of domineering over animals. It seems almost needless to say how easy the transition is, in such cases, should opportunity offer, from tyranny over the brute slave, to tyranny over the human being. There are slave-holders in the family and in the school, as well as elsewhere. It is the SPIRIT of a person which makes him either a tyrant or slave-holder. And let us beware how we foster this spirit in the children whom God has given us.

# CHAPTER XI.

## AMUSEMENTS.

Universal need of amusements. Why so necessary. Error of schools. Error of families. Infant schools, as often conducted, particularly injurious. Lessons, or tasks, should be short. Mistakes of some manual labor schools. Of particular amusements in the nursery. With small wooden cubes—pictures—shuttlecock—the rocking horse—tops and marbles—backgammon—checkers—morrice—dice—nine-pins—skipping the rope—trundling the hoop—playing at ball—kites—skating and swimming—dissected maps—black boards—elements of letters—dissected pictures.

However heterodox the concession may be, I am one of those who believe amusements of some sort or other to be universally necessary. Indeed I cannot possibly conceive of an individual in health, whatever may be the age, sex, condition, or employment, who does not need them, in a greater or less degree.

Now if by the term amusement, I merely meant employment, nobody would probably differ from me—at least in theory. Every one is ready to admit the importance of being constantly employed. A mind unemployed is a VACANT mind. And a vacant or idle mind is "the devil's work-shop;" so says the proverb.

By amusement, however, I mean something more than mere employment; for the more constantly an adult individual is employed, the greater, generally, is his demand for amusement. Indolent persons have less need of being amused than others; but perhaps there are few if any persons to be found, who are so indolent as not to think continually, on one subject or another. And it is this constant thinking, more than anything else, that creates the necessity of which I am speaking. The mere drudge, whether biped or quadruped—he, I mean, whose thinking powers are scarcely alive—has little need of the relief which is afforded by amusement.

The young of all animals—man among the rest—appear to have such an instinctive fondness for amusement, that so long as they are unrestrained, they seldom need any urging on this point. In regard to *quality*, the case is somewhat different. In this respect, most children require attention and restraint; and some of them a great deal of it.

But what is the nature of the amusement which adults—nay, mankind generally—require? I answer, it is relief from the employment of thinking. For it is not that mankind do not really think at all, that moralists complain so loudly. When they tell us that men will not think, they mean that they will not think as rational beings. They think, indeed; and so do the ox, and the horse, and the dog, and the elephant—but not as rational men ought to do; and this it is that constitutes the burden of complaint. But you will probably find few persons belonging to the human species who do not think constantly, at least while awake; and whose mental powers do not become fatigued, and demand relief in amusement.

Children's minds are so soon wearied by a continuous train of thinking, even on topics which are pleasing to them, that they can seldom he brought to give their attention to a single subject long at once. They require almost incessant change; both for the sake of relief, and to amuse for the *sake* of amusement. And it is, to my own mind, one of the most striking proofs of Infinite Wisdom in the creation of the human mind, that it has, during infancy, such an irresistible tendency to amusement.

How greatly do they err, who grudge children, especially very young children, the time which, in obedience to the dictates of their nature, they are so fond of spending in sports and gambols! How much more rational would it be to encourage and direct them in their amusements! And how exceedingly unwise is the practice, whenever and wherever it exists, of confining them to school rooms and benches, not only for hours, but for whole half days at once.

If individuals and circumstances were everywhere combined, with the special purpose to oppose the intentions of nature respecting the human being, at every step of his progress from the cradle to maturity, and from maturity to the grave, I hardly know how they could contrive to accomplish such a purpose more effectually than it is at present accomplished. But it is proper that I should here explain a little.

All our family arrangements tend to repress amusement. Everything is contrived to facilitate business—especially the business or employments of adults. The child is hardly regarded as a human being,—certainly not as a *perfect* being. He is considered as a mere fragment; or to change the figure, as a plant too young to be of any real service to mankind, because too young to bear any of its appropriate fruits. Whereas, in my opinion, both infancy and childhood, at every stage, should bring forth their appropriate fruits. In other words, the child of the most tender years should be regarded as a whole, and not as the mere fragment of a being; as a perfect member of a family—occupying a full and complete, only a more limited sphere than older members: and all the rules and regulations and arrangements of the family should have a reference to this point. So long as a child is reckoned to be a mere cipher in creation, or at most, as of no more practical importance, till the arrival of his twenty-first birth day, or some other equally arbitrary period, than our domestic animals—that is, of just sufficient consequence to be fed, and caressed, and fondled, and made a pet of—so long will our arrangements be made with reference to the comfort and happiness of adults. There may indeed be here and there a child's chair, or a child's carriage, or newspaper, or book; but there will seldom be, except by stealth, any free juvenile conversation at the table or the fireside. Here the child must sit as a blank or cypher, to ruminate on the past, or to receive half formed and passive impressions from the present.

The arrangements of the infant school, also, seem designed for the same purpose—to repress as much as possible the infantile desire for amusement. Not that this was their original, nor that it now is their legitimate intention. Their legitimate object is, or should be, not to develope the intellect by over-working the tender brain, but to promote cheerfulness and health and love and happiness, by well contrived amusements, conducted as much as possible in the open air; and by unremitting efforts to elicit and direct the affections.

Infant schools should repress rather than encourage the hard study of books. Lessons at this age should be drawn chiefly from objects in the garden, the field, and the grove; from the flower, the plant, the tree, the brook, the bird, the beast, the worm, the fly, the human body—the sun, or the visible heavens. These lessons, whether given by the parent, as constituting a part of the family arrangements, or by the infant or primary school teacher, should, it is true, be regarded for the time being as study, but they should never be long; and they should be frequently relieved by the most free and unrestrained pastimes and gambols of the young on the green grass, or beside the rippling stream, uninfluenced, or at least unrepressed, by those who are set over them.

The public or common school, overlooking as it does any direct attempts to make provision for the amusement of the pupils, even during the scanty recess that is afforded them once in three hours, would appear to a stranger on this planet, at first sight, to be designed as much as possible to defeat every intention of nature with reference to the growth of the human frame. For we may often travel many hundred miles and not see so much as an enclosed play ground; and never perhaps any direct provision for particular and more favorable amusements.

I might speak of other schools and places of resort for children, and proceed to show how all our arrangements appear to be the offspring of a species of utilitarianism which rejects every sport whose value cannot be estimated in dollars and cents. I might even refer to those schools of our country where these ultra utilitarian notions are carried to an extent which excludes amusing conversation or reading even during meal-time; and devotes the hours which were formerly spent in recreation, to manual labor of some productive kind or other.—But I forbear. Enough has been said to illustrate the position I have taken, that there is in vogue a system which bears the marks of having been contrived, if not by the enemies of our race, either openly or covertly, at least by those whom ignorance renders scarcely less at war with the general happiness.

Now I would not deny nor attempt to deny that change of occupation of body or mind is of itself an amusement, and one too of great value. Undoubtedly it is so. To some children, studies of every kind are an amusement; and there are few indeed to whom none are so. Labor, with many, when alternated with study, is amusing. And yet, after all, unless such labors are performed in company, where light and cheerful conversation is sure to keep the mind away from the subjects about which it has just been engaged, I am afraid that the purposes for which amusements were designed, are very far from being *all* secured.

But perhaps I am dwelling too long on the general principle that people of every age, and children in particular, need, and must have amusements, whether they are of a productive kind or not; and that it is very far from being sufficient, were it either practicable or desirable, to turn all study and labor into amusement. [Footnote: I will even say, more distinctly than I have already done, that however popular the contrary opinion may be, neither study nor work ought to be regarded as mere amusement. I would, it is true, take every possible pains to render both work and study agreeable; but I would at the same time have it distinctly understood, that one of them is by no means the other; that, on the contrary, work is *work*—study, *study*—and amusement, *amusement*.] My business is with those who direct the first dawnings of affection and intellect. Principles are by no means of less importance on this account; but the limits of a work for young mothers do not admit of anything more than a brief discussion of their importance.

I will now proceed to speak of some of the more common amusements of the nursery.

I have seen very young children sit on the floor and amuse themselves for nearly half an hour together, with piling up and taking down small wooden cubes, of different sizes. Some of them, instead of being cubes, however, may be of the shape of bricks. Their ingenuity, while they are scarcely a year or two old, in erecting houses, temples, churches, &c., is sometimes surprising. Girls as well as boys seem to be greatly amused with this form of exercise; and both seem to be little less gratified in destroying than in rearing their lilliputian edifices.

Next to the latter kind of amusement, is the viewing of pictures. It is surprising at what an early age children may be taught to notice miniature representations of objects; living objects especially. Representations of the works of art should come in a little later than those of things in nature. I know a father who prepares volumes of pictures, solely for this purpose; though he usually regards them not only as a source of amusement to children, but as a medium of instruction.

Battledoor or shuttlecock may be taught to children of both sexes very early; and it affords a healthy and almost untiring source of amusement. It gives activity as well as strength to the muscles or moving powers, and has many other important advantages. There is some danger, according to Dr. Pierson [Footnote: See his Lecture before the American Institute of Instruction] of distorting the spine by playing at shuttlecock too frequently and too long; but this will seldom be the case with little children in the nursery. Neither shuttlecock nor any other amusement will secure their attention long enough to injure them very much.

Perhaps this exercise comes nearer to my ideas of a perfect amusement than almost any which could be named. The mind is agreeably occupied, without being fatigued; and if the amusements are proportioned to the age and strength of the child, there is very little fatigue of the body. It gives, moreover, great practical accuracy to the eye and to the hand.

A rocking-horse is much recommended for the nursery. I have had no opportunity for observing the effects of this kind of amusement; but if it is one half as valuable as some suppose, I should be inclined to recommend it. But I am opposed to fostering in the rider lessons of cruelty, by arming him with whips and spurs. If the young are ever to learn to ride, on a living horse, the exercises of the rocking-horse will, most certainly, be a sort of preparation for the purpose.

Tops and marbles afford a great deal of rational amusement to the young; and of a very useful kind, too. Spinning a top is second to no exercise which I have yet mentioned, unless it is playing at shuttlecock.

Dr. Dewees recommends a small backgammon table, with men, but without dice. He says, also, that "children, as soon as they are capable of comprehending the subject, should be taught draughts or checkers. This game is not only highly amusing, but also very instructive." In another place he heaps additional encomiums upon the game of checkers. "It becomes a source of endless amusement," he says, "as it never tires, but always instructs." Of exercises which instruct, however, as well as amuse, I shall speak presently.

The amusements called "morrice," "fox and geese," &c., with which some of the children of almost every neighborhood are more or less acquainted, are of the same general character and tendency as checkers. So is a play, sometimes, but very improperly, called dice, in which two parties play with a small bundle of wooden pins, not unlike knitting pins in shape, but shorter.

The writer to whom I have referred above recommends nine-pins and balls of proper size, as highly useful both for diversion and exercise. If they can be used without leading to bad habits and bad associations, I think they may be useful.

For girls, who demand a great deal more of exercise, both within doors and without, skipping the rope is an excellent amusement. So also is swinging. Both of these exercises may be used either out of doors, or in the nursery.

Trundling a hoop I have always regarded as an amusing out-of-door exercise; and I am not sorry when I sometimes see girls, as well as boys, engaged in it, under the eye of their mothers and teachers.

Playing ball, of which there are many different games, and flying kites, employ a large proportion if not all of the muscles of the body, in such a manner as is likely to confirm the strength, and greatly improve the health. The same may be said of skating in the winter, and swimming in the summer. But these last are exercises over which the mother cannot, ordinarily, have very much control.

Under the head of amusements, it only remains for me to speak of a few juvenile employments of a mixed nature. Of these I shall treat very briefly, as they are a branch of the subject which does not necessarily come within the compass of my present plan. They are exercises, too, which should more properly come under the head of Infantile Instruction.

Dissected maps afford children of every age a great fund of amusement; but much caution is necessary, with those that are very young, not to discourage or confound them by showing them too many at once. Thus if we cut in pieces the map of one of the smaller United States, at the county lines, or the whole United States, at the state lines, it is quite as many divisions as they can manage. Cut up as large a state, even, as Pennsylvania or New York is, into counties, and try to lead them to amuse themselves by putting together so large a number, many of which must inevitably very closely resemble each other, and it is ten to one but you bewilder, and even perplex and discourage them. The same results would follow from cutting up even the whole of a large county, or a small state, into towns. I have usually begun with little children, by requiring them to put together the eight counties of the small state of Connecticut. In this case the counties are not only few, but there is a very striking difference in their shape.

A black board and a piece of chalk, along with a little ingenuity on the part of the mother, will furnish the child with an almost endless variety of amusement. Let him attempt to imitate almost any object which interests him, whether among the works of nature or art. However rude his pictures may be, do not laugh at, but on the contrary, endeavor to encourage him. He may also be permitted to imitate letters and figures. The elements of letters, too, both printed and written, may be given him, and he may be required to put them together. Dissected pictures, as well as dissected maps and letters, are useful, and to most children, very acceptable.

In short, the devices of an ingenious, thinking mother, for the amusement of her very young children, are almost endless; and the great danger is, that when a mother once enters deeply into the spirit of these exercises, she will substitute them for those much more healthy ones which have been already mentioned, such as require muscular activity, or may be performed in the open air.

# CHAPTER XII.

## CRYING.

Its importance. Danger of repressing a tendency to cry. Anecdote from Dr. Rush. Physiology of crying. Folly of attempting wholly to suppress it.

"Crying," says Dr. Dewees, "should be looked upon as an exercise of much importance;" and he is sustained in this view by many eminent medical writers.

But people generally think otherwise. Nothing is more common than the idea that to cry is unbecoming; and children are everywhere taught, when they suffer pain, to brave it out, and *not cry*. Such a direction—to say nothing of its tendency to encourage hypocrisy—is wholly unphilosophical. The following anecdote may serve in part to illustrate my meaning. It is said to have been related by Dr. Rush.

A gentleman in South Carolina was about to undergo a very painful surgical operation. He had imbibed the idea that it was beneath the dignity of a man ever to say or do anything expressive of pain. He therefore refused to submit to the usual precaution of securing the hands and feet by bandages, declaring to his surgeon that he had nothing to fear from his being untied, for he would not move a muscle of his body. He kept his word, it is true; but he died instantly after the operation, from apoplexy.

There is very little doubt, in the mind of any physiologist, in regard to the cause of apoplexy in this case; and that it might have been prevented by the relief which is always afforded by groans and tears.

It is, I believe, very generally known, that in the profoundest grief, people do not, and cannot shed tears; and that when the *latter* begin to flow, it affords immediate relief.

I do not undertake to argue from this, that crying is so important, either to the young or the old, that it is ever worth while to excite or continue it by artificial means; or that a habit of crying, so easily and readily acquired by the young, is not to be guarded against as a serious, evil. My object was first to show the folly of those who denounce all crying, and secondly, to point out some of its advantages—in the hope of preventing parents from going to that extreme which borders upon stoicism.

One of the most intelligent men I ever knew, frequently made it his boast that he neither laughed nor cried on any occasion; and on being told that both laughing and crying were physiologically useful, he only ridiculed the sentiment.

Crying is useful to very young infants, because it favors the passage of blood in their lungs, where it had not before been accustomed to travel, and where its motion is now indispensable. And it not only promotes the circulation of the blood, but expands the air-cells of the lungs, and thus helps forward that great change, by which the dark-colored impure blood of the veins is changed at once into pure blood, and thus rendered fit to nourish the system, and sustain life.

But this is not all. Crying strengthens the lungs themselves. It does this by expanding the little air-cells of which I have just spoken, and not only accustoms them to being stretched, at a period, of all others, the most favorable for this purpose, but frees them at the same time from mucus, and other injurious accumulations.

They, therefore, who oppose an infant's crying, know not what they do. So far is it from being hurtful to the child, that its occasional recurrence is, as we have already seen, positively useful. Some practitioners of medicine, in some of the more trying situations in which human nature can be placed, even encourage their patients to suffer tears to flow, as a means of relief.

Infants, it should also be recollected, have no other language by which to express their wants and feelings, than sighs and tears. Crying is not always an expression of positive pain; it sometimes indicates hunger and thirst, and sometimes the want of a change of posture. This last consideration deserves great attention, and all the inconveniences of crying ought to be borne cheerfully, for the sake of having the little sufferer remind us when nature demands a change of position. No child ought to be permitted to remain in one position longer than two hours, even while sleeping; nor half that time, while awake; and if nurses and mothers will overlook this matter, as they often do, it is a favorable circumstance that the child should remind them of it.

Crying has been called the "waste gate" of the human system; the door of escape to that excess of excitability which sometimes prevails, especially among children and nervous adults. To all such persons it is healthy—most undoubtedly so; nor do I know that its occasional recurrence is injurious to any adult—a fastidious public sentiment to the contrary notwithstanding.

Some have supposed, that what is here said will be construed by the young mother into a license to suffer her child to cry unnecessarily. Perhaps, say they, she is a laboring woman, and wishes to be at work. Well, she lays down her child in the cradle, or on the bed, and goes to her work. Presently the child, becoming wet perhaps, begins to cry, as well he might. But, instead of going to him and taking care of him, she continues at her employment; and when one remonstrates against her conduct as cruelty, she pleads the authority of the author of the "Young Mother."

All this may happen; but if it should, I am not answerable for it. I have insisted strongly on guarding the child against wet clothing, and on watching him with the utmost care to prevent all real suffering. Mothers, like the specimen here given, if they happen to have a little sensibility to suffering, and not much love of their offspring, generally know of a shorter way to quiet their infants and procure time to work, than that which is here mentioned. They have nothing to do but to give them some cordial or elixir, whose basis is opium. Startle not, reader, at the statement;—this abominable practice is followed by many a female who claims the sacred name of mother. And many a wretch has thus, in her ignorance, indolence or avarice, slowly destroyed her children!

I repeat, therefore, that I do not think my remarks on crying are necessarily liable to abuse; though I am not sure that there are not a few individuals to be found who may apply them in the manner above mentioned—an application, however, which is as far removed from the original intention of the author, as can possibly be conceived.

# CHAPTER XIII.

## LAUGHING.

"Laugh and be fat." Laughing is healthy. A common error. Monastic notions yet too prevalent on this subject.

Laughing, like crying, has a good effect on the infantile lungs; nor is it less salutary in other respects. "Laugh and be fat," an old adage, has its meaning, and also its philosophy.

There is an excess, however, to which laughing, no less than crying, may be carried, and which we cannot too carefully avoid. But how little to be envied—how much to be pitied—are they who consider it a weakness and a sin to laugh, and in the plenitude of their wisdom, tell us that *the Saviour of mankind never laughed*. When I hear this last assertion, I am always ready to ask, whether the individual who makes it has read a new revelation or a new gospel; for certainly none of the sacred books which I have seen give us any such information.

But I will not dwell here. The common notion on this subject, if not ridiculous, is certainly strange. I will only add, that, come into vogue as it might have done, there is no opinion more unfounded than the very general one among adults, that children should be uniformly grave; and that just in proportion as they laugh and appear frolicsome, just in the same proportion are they out of the way, and deserving of reprehension.

It is strange that it should be so, but I have seen many parents who were miserable because their children were sportive and joyful. Oh, when will the days of monkish sadness and austerity be over; and the public sentiment in the christian world get right on this subject!

# CHAPTER XIV.

## SLEEP.

General remarks. Hints to fathers.—SEC. 1. Proper hours for repose. Dark rooms. Noise.—SEC. 2. Place for sleeping. Sleeping alone—reasons.—SEC. 3. Purity of the air in sleeping rooms.—SEC. 4. The bed. Objections to feathers. Other materials.—SEC. 5. The covering of beds. Covering the head.—SEC. 6. Night Dresses. Robes.—SEC. 7. Posture of the body in sleep.—SEC. 8. State of the mind.—SEC. 9. Quality of sleep.—SEC. 10. Quantity of sleep.

Not a few persons consider all rules relative to sleep as utterly futile. They regard it as so much of a natural or animal process, that if we are let alone we shall seldom err, at any age, respecting it. Rules on the subject, above all, they regard as wholly misplaced.

Those who entertain such views, would do well, in order to be consistent, to go a little farther; and as breathing and eating and drinking—nay, even *thinking*—are natural processes, deny the utility of all rules respecting *them* also. Perhaps they would do well, moreover, to deny that rules of any sort are valuable. But would not this have the effect to bar the door perpetually against all human improvement? Would it not be equivalent to saying, to a half-civilized, because only half-christianized community—Go on with your barbarous customs, and your uncleanly and unthinking habits, forever?

But I have not so learned human nature. I regard man as susceptible of endless progression. And I know of no way in which more rapid progress can be made, than by enlightening young mothers on subjects which pertain to our physical nature, and the means of physical improvement. Not for the *sake* of that perishable part of man, the frame, but because it is nearly in vain to attempt to improve the mind and heart, without due attention to the frame-work, to which mind and heart, for the present, are appended, and most intimately related.

Let it be left to fathers to study the improvement of hounds and horses and cattle, and at the same time to think themselves above the concerns of the nursery. We may, indeed, read of a Cato once in three thousand years, who was in the habit of quitting all other business in order to be present when the nurse washed and rubbed his child. But our passion for gain, in the present age, is so much more absorbing and soul-destroying than the passion for military glory, that we cannot expect many Catos. Oh no. All, or nearly all, must devolve on the mother. The father has no time to attend to his children! What belongs to the mother, if she can be duly awakened, may be at least *half* done; what belongs to the father, must, I fear, be left undone.

I am accustomed to regard every day—even of the infant—as a miniature life. I am, moreover, accustomed to consider mental and bodily vigor, not only for each separate day, but for life's whole day, as greatly influenced by the circumstances of sleep; the HOUR, PLACE, PURITY OF THE AIR, THE BED, THE COVERING, DRESS, POSTURE, STATE OF THE MIND, QUALITY, QUANTITY, AND DURATION.

## SEC. 1. *Hour for Repose.*

Generally speaking, the night is the appropriate season for repose; but in early infancy, it is *every* hour. I have already spoken of the vast amount of sleep which the new-born infant requires, as well as of many other circumstances connected with it, requiring our attention. Suffer me, however, to enlarge, at the risk of a little repetition.

What time the infant is awake, should be during the day. It is of very great importance, in the formation of good habits, that he should be undressed and put to bed, at evening, with as much regularity as if be had not slept during the day for a single moment. It is also important that he be permitted to sleep during the whole night, as uninterruptedly as possible; and that when he is aroused, to have his position or diapers changed, or to receive food, it should be done with little parade and noise, and with as little light as possible. All persons, old as well as young, sleep more quietly in a dark room, than in one where a light is burning.

I am well aware that the course here recommended, may be carried to an excess which will utterly defeat the object intended, since there are children to be found, who are so trained in this respect, that the lightest tread upon the floor will awake, and perhaps frighten them. But this is an excess which is not required. All that is necessary during the night, is a reasonable degree of silence, in order to induce the habit of continued rest, if possible. In the day time, on the contrary, fatigue will impel a child to sleep occasionally, even in the midst of noise. I am not sure that the habit of sleeping in the midst of noise is not worth a little pains on the part of the mother. Nor is it improbable that a habit of this kind, once acquired by the infant, might ultimately be extended to the night, so that over-caution, even in regard to that season, might gradually be laid aside.

Dr. North, a distinguished medical practitioner in Hartford, Conn., confirms the foregoing sentiments; and adds, that he deems it an imperious duty of those parents who wish well to their infants, to form in them the habit of sleeping when fatigued, whether the room be quiet or noisy. With his children, no cradles or opiates are needed or used.

### SEC. 2. *Place.*

For some time after its birth, the infant should sleep near its mother, though not in the same bed. The bedstead should be of the usual height of bedsteads, and should be enclosed with a railing sufficient to secure the infant from falling out, but not of such a structure as to hinder, in any degree, a free circulation of the air.

The reasons why a child ought to sleep alone, and not with the mother or nurse, are numerous; but the following are the principal;

1. The heat accumulated by the bodies of the mother and child both, is often too great for health.

2. The air is too impure. I have already spoken of the change in the purity of the air which is produced by breathing in it. It is bad enough for two adults to sleep in the same bed, breathing over and over again the impure air, as they must do more or less, even if the bed is very large;—but it is still

worse for infants. Their lungs demand atmospheric air in its utmost purity; and if denied it, they must eventually suffer.

3. But besides the change of the air by breathing, the surface of the body is perpetually changing it in the same manner, as was stated in the chapter on Ventilation. Now a child will almost inevitably breathe a stream of this bad air, as it issues from the bed; and what is still worse, it is very apt, in spite of every precaution, to get its head covered up with the clothes, where it can hardly breathe anything else. This, if frequently repeated, is slow but certain death;—as much so as if the child were to drink poison in moderate quantities.

Let me not be told that this is an exaggeration; that thousands of mothers make it a point to cover up the beads of their infants; and that notwithstanding this, they are as healthy as the infants of their neighbors. I have not said that they would droop and die while infants. The fumes of lead, which is a certain poison, may be inhaled, and yet the child or adult who inhales them may live on, in tolerable health, for many years. But suffer he must, in the end, in spite of every effort and every hope. So must the child, whose head is covered habitually with the bed clothing, where it is compelled to breathe not only the air spoiled by its own skin, but also that which is spoiled by the much larger surface of body of the mother or nurse.

But I have proof on this subject. Friedlander, in his "Physical Education," says expressly, that in Great Britain alone, between the years 1686 and 1800, no less than 40,000 children died in consequence of this practice of allowing them to sleep near their nurses. I was at first disposed to doubt the accuracy of this most remarkable statement. But when I consider the respectability of the authority from which it emanated, and that it is only about 350 a year for that great empire, I cannot doubt that the estimate is substantially correct. What a sacrifice at the shrine of ignorance and folly!

It should be added, in this place, both to confirm the foregoing sentiment, and to show that British mothers and nurses are not alone, that Dr. Dewees has witnessed, in the circle of his practice, four deaths from the same cause. If every physician in the United States has met with as many cases of the kind, in proportion to his practice, as Dr. D., the evil is about as great in this country as Dr. F. says it is in Great Britain.

If a child sleeps alone, it cannot of course be liable to as much suffering of this kind as if it slept with another person; though much precaution will still be necessary to keep its head uncovered, and prevent its inhaling air spoiled by its own lungs and skin.

4. There is one more evil which will be avoided by having a child sleep alone. Many a mother has seriously injured her child by pressure. I do not here allude to those monsters in human nature, whose besotted habits have been the frequent cause of the suffocation and death of their offspring, but to the more careful and tender mother, who would sooner injure herself than her own child. Such mothers, even, have been known to dislocate or fracture a limb![Footnote: There may be instances where the debility of an infant will be so great that the mother or a nurse must sleep with it, to keep it warm. But such cases of disease are very rare.]

To cap the climax of error in this matter, some mothers allow their infants to lie on their arm, as a pillow. This practice not only exposes them to all or nearly all the evils which have been mentioned, but to one more; viz. the danger of being thrown from the bed.

A young mother, with whom I was well acquainted, was sleeping one night with her infant on her arm, when she made a sudden and rather violent effort to turn in the bed, in doing which she threw the child upon the floor with such violence as to fracture its little skull, and cause its death.

Enough, I trust, has now been said to convince every reasonable young mother, where absolute poverty does not preclude comfort and health, that her child ought never to be permitted to sleep in the same bed with her; but that it should be placed on a bedstead by itself at a short distance from her, and properly guarded from accidents—and above all, from inhaling impure air.

At a suitable age, a child may be removed from the nursery to a separate chamber. Here, if the circumstances permit, it should still sleep by itself; and if the bedstead be somewhat lower than ordinary, and the room be not too small, it will need no watching.

Perhaps this may be the proper place to say that there are more reasons than one—and some of them are of a moral nature, too—why a child should continue to sleep alone, after it leaves the nursery. Nor is it sufficient to prohibit its sleeping with younger persons, and yet crowd it into the bed with an aged grandfather or grandmother, or with both. There is no excuse for a course like this, except the iron hand of necessity. And even then, I should prefer to have a child of mine sleep on the hard floor, at least during the summer season, rather than with an aged person.

Let it not be supposed I have imbibed the fashionable idea that it is *peculiarly* unhealthy for the young to sleep with the old. I know this doctrine has many learned advocates. And yet I doubt its correctness. I believe that the manners and habits of the old may injure the young who sleep with them, and I know that they render the air impure, like other people. But I cannot see why the mere circumstance of their being *old* should be a source of unhealthiness to their younger bed-fellows. Still I say, that there are reasons enough against the practice I am opposing, without this.

Some parents allow dogs and cats to sleep with children. Others have a prejudice against cats, but not against dogs. The truth is, that they both contaminate the air by respiration and perspiration, in the same manner that adults do. And aside from the fact that they are often infested by lice and other insects, and addicted to uncleanly habits, they ought always to be excluded, and with iron bars and bolts, if necessary, from the beds of children. But of this, too, I have treated elsewhere.

## SEC. 3. *Purity of the Air.*

The general importance of pure air has been mentioned. I have spoken of the elements of the atmosphere in which we live, of the manner in which it may be vitiated, and the consequences to health. I have shown—perhaps at sufficient length—the impropriety of washing, drying, and ironing clothes in the room where a child is kept; of cooking in the room, especially on a stove; of suffering the floor or clothes, particularly those of the child, to remain long wet, in the room; of smoking tobacco, using spirits, burning oil with too long a wick, &c.

All which has thus been said of the purity of the air of the nursery generally, is applicable to that of all sleeping rooms. It is an important point gained, when we can secure a nursery with folding doors in the centre, so as, when we please, to make two rooms of it. In that case, the division in which the bed is, can be completely ventilated a little before night, and thus be comparatively pure for the reception of both the mother and the child.

Shall the windows and doors where a child sleeps, be kept closed; or shall they be suffered to remain open a part or the whole of the night? This must be determined by circumstances. If there are no doors but such as communicate with apartments whose air is equally impure with that in which the child is, it is preferable to keep them closed. If the windows cannot be opened without exposing the child to a current of air, it is perhaps the less of two evils, not to open them.

But we are not usually driven to such extremities. In some instances, windows are constructed—and all of them ought to be—so that they can be lowered from the top. When this is not the case, something can be placed before the window to break the current, so that it need not fall directly upon the child. Closing the blinds will partially effect this, where blinds exist.

I have known many an individual who was in the habit of sleeping with his windows open during the whole year, and without any obvious evil consequences. Dr. Gregory was of this habit. But if adults—not trained to it—can acquire such a habit with impunity, with how much more safety could children be trained to it from the very first year. Macnish says, "there can be no doubt that a gentle current pervading our sleeping apartments, is in the highest degree ESSENTIAL TO HEALTH."

This consideration—I mean the impurity of sleeping rooms, even after every precaution has been used to keep them ventilated—affords one of the strongest inducements to going abroad early in the morning (especially when there is no other room which either adults or children can occupy) while the nursery or chamber is aired and ventilated. The utility of *rising* early, I hope no one can doubt; but some have doubts of the propriety of going abroad, till the dew has "passed away." Such should be reminded, by the foregoing train of remarks, that early walking may be a choice of evils; and that if it *is* on the whole advantageous to adults, it cannot be less so to children. And as soon as the sun has chased away the vapors of the night, if the weather is tolerable, most children should be carried abroad.

### SEC. 4. *The Bed.*

This should never be of feathers. There are many reasons for this prohibition, especially to the feeble.

1. They are too warm. Infants should by all means be kept warm enough, as I have all along insisted. But excess of heat excites or stimulates the skin, causing an unnatural degree of perspiration, and thus inducing weakness or debility.

2. When we first enter a room in which there is a feather bed which has been occupied during the night, we are struck with the offensive smell of the air. This is owing to a variety of causes; one of which probably is, that beds of this kind are better adapted to absorb and retain the effluvia of our bodies. But let the causes be what they may, the effects ought, if possible, to be avoided; for both experience and authority combine to pronounce them very injurious.

3. Feather beds—if used in the nursery—will inevitably discharge more or less of dust and down; both of which are injurious to the tender lungs of the infant.

Mattresses are better for persons of every age, than soft feather beds. They may be made of horse hair or moss; but hair is the best. If the mattress does not appear to be warm enough for the very young infant, a blanket may be spread over it. Dr. Dewees says that in case mattresses cannot be had, "the sacking bottom" may be substituted, or "even the floor;" at least in warm weather: "for almost anything," he adds, "is preferable to feathers."

I have no hostility to soft beds, especially for young children and feeble adults, could softness be secured without much heat and relaxation of the system. On the contrary, it is certainly desirable, in itself, to have the bed so soft that as large a proportion of the surface of the body may rest on it as possible. But I consider hardness as a much smaller evil than feathers.

It is worthy of remark how generally physicians, for the last hundred years, have recommended hard beds, especially straw beds or hair mattresses, to their more feeble and delicate patients. This fact might at least quiet our apprehensions in regard to their tendency on those who are accustomed to them in early infancy.

Some writers on these subjects appear to doubt whether, after all that they say, they shall have much influence on mothers in inducing them to give up feather beds for their infants. But they need not be so faithless. Multitudes have already been reformed by their writings; and multitudes larger still would be so, could they gain access to them. It is a most serious evil that they are often so written and published that comparatively few mothers will ever possess them.

The pillow, as well as the bed, should be rather hard; and its thickness should be much less than is usual, or we shall do mischief by bending the neck, and thus compressing the vessels, and obstructing the circulation of the blood. But on this subject I will say more, when I come to treat on "Posture."

The child's bed should not be placed near the wall, on account of dampness. There is also, during the summer, another reason. Should lightning strike the house, it will be much more apt to injure those who are near the wall than other persons; as it seldom leaves the wall to pass over the central part of the room.

Curtains are not only useless, but injurious. They prevent a free circulation of the air. Everything which has this tendency must be studiously guarded against, in the management of infants.

Nothing is more injurious to the old or the young than damp beds and damp covering. It behoves, especially, all those who have the care of infants, to see that everything about their beds is thoroughly dry. The walls and clothes should also be dry; and wet clothes should never be hung up in the room. By neglecting these precautions, colds, rheumatisms, inflammations, fevers, consumptions, and death, may ensue. Many a person loses his health, and not a few their lives, in this way. The author of this work was once thrown into a fever from such a cause.

Warming the bed is, in all cases, a bad practice. While in the nursery, if the air be kept at a proper temperature, there will be no need of it; after the child is assigned to a separate chamber, its enervating tendency would result in more evil than good. It is better to let the bed became gradually heated by the body, in a natural and healthy way.

No person, and above all, no infant, should be suffered to sleep in a bed that has been recently occupied by the sick. The bed and all the clothes should first be thoroughly aired. Could we see with our eyes at once, how rapidly these bodies of ours fill the air, and even the beds we sleep in, with carbonic acid and other hurtful gases and impurities, even while in health, but much more so in sickness, we should be cautious of exposing the lungs of the tender infant, in such an atmosphere, until everything had been properly cleansed, and the apartments properly ventilated.

### SEC. 5. *The Covering.*

The covering of the bed should be sufficiently warm, but never any warmer than is absolutely necessary to protect the child from chilliness. The lightest covering which will secure this object is the best. Perhaps there is nothing in use that, with so little weight, secures so much heat as what are called "comfortables."

The clothes should not be "tucked up" at the sides and foot of the bed with too much care and exactness. For when the bed is once warmed thoroughly with the child's body, the admission of a little fresh air into it, when he elevates or otherwise moves his limbs, can do no harm, but *may* do much of good, in the way of ventilation. I deem it important, moreover, to inure children very early to little partial exposures of this kind.

Those mothers who, from over-tenderness, and want of correct information on the subject, pursue a contrary course, and consider it as almost certain death to have a particle of fresh air reach the bodies of their infants during their slumbers, are generally sure to outwit themselves, and defeat their very intentions. For by being thus tender of their children, it often turns out that whenever the mother is ill, or when on any other account she ceases to watch over them—and such times must, in general, sooner or later come—they are much more liable to take cold or sustain other injury, should they be exposed, than if they had been treated more rationally.

I knew a mother who would not trust her children to take care of their own beds on retiring to rest, as long as they remained in her house, even though they were twenty or thirty years old. But they had no better or firmer constitutions than the other children of the same neighborhood.

Hardly anything can be more injurious than covering the head with the bed clothes; and yet some mothers and nurses cover, in this way, not only their own heads, but those of their children. I have elsewhere shown how impure the air is, which is imprisoned under the bed clothes. I hope those mothers who are willing to destroy *themselves* by covering up their heads while they sleep, will at least have mercy on their unoffending infants.

### SEC. 6. *Night Dresses.*

The grand rule on this point is, to wear as little dress during sleep as possible. Some mothers not only suffer their infants to sleep in the same shirt, cap, and stockings that they have worn during the day, but add a night gown to the rest. No cap should be worn during the night, any more than in the day time. Or if the foolish practice has been adopted for the day, it should be discontinued at night. It is enough for those adults whose long hair would otherwise be dishevelled, to wear night caps, and subject themselves, as they inevitably do, to catarrh and periodical headache. Children's heads should have nothing on them by night; nor even by day, except to defend them from the rain or the hot rays of the sun.

The stockings, too, should be wholly laid aside at night, unless in the case of those who are feeble, apt to have their feet cold, or particularly liable to bowel complaints. Such may be allowed to sleep in their stockings, but not in those which have been worn all the day.

Indeed, neither children nor adults should ever wear a single garment in the night which they have worn during the day. The reason is, that there are too many causes of impurity in operation while we sleep, without our wearing the clothes in which we have been perspiring during the day-time—and which must be already more or less filled with the effluvia of our bodies.

It is a very easy thing to have a loose night gown to supply the place of the shirt we have worn during the day; and if nothing else is convenient, a spare shirt will answer. But both a night gown and shirt should never be admitted, especially in warm weather. The garment to supply the place of the shirt during the night, may be of calico in the summer, and of flannel in the winter.

The collar and wristbands of this night dress should be loose; and the whole garment should be large and long. No article of dress should ever press upon our bodies, so as in the least to impede the circulation; and for this reason it is, that writers on physical education have inveighed so much against cravats, straps, garters, &c. This caution, so important to all, is doubly so to young mothers, on whom devolves the management of the tender infant.

When the child has been perspiring freely during the evening, just before he is undressed, or when he has just been subjected to the warm bath, it may be well to use a little care in undressing and exchanging clothes, to prevent taking cold;—though it should ever be remembered, that those children who are managed on a rational system will bear slight exposures with far more safety, than they who have been managed at random—sometimes, indeed, with great tenderness, but at others, wholly neglected.

## SEC. 7. *Posture of the Body.*

In early infancy, children who are not stuffed rather than fed, may occasionally be permitted to sleep on their backs, especially if they incline to do so. But it will be well to encourage them to sleep on one side, as soon as you can without great inconvenience.

The right side, as a general rule, is preferable; because the stomach, which lies towards the left side, is thus left uncompressed, and digestion undisturbed. I would not, however, require a child to lie always on the right side, but would occasionally change his position, lest he should become unable to sleep at all, except in a particular manner.

I have said elsewhere, that the head ought to be a little raised, especially if the child is liable to diseases of the brain. But this remark, rather hastily thrown out, requires explanation.

There is so much blood sent by the heart to the head and upper parts of the system of infants, as to predispose those parts, especially the brain, to disease. In a horizontal position of the body, there is more blood sent to the brain than when the body is erect. This will show the reader, at once, that if the infant is peculiarly exposed to diseases of the brain—and it certainly is so—he ought to remain in a horizontal posture as little as possible, except during sleep; and that even then it is desirable to make his bed in such a manner as to elevate the head and shoulders as much as we can without compressing the lungs, or obstructing the circulation in the neck.

I recommend, therefore, to raise the head of an infant's bedstead a little higher than the foot; though not so much as to incline him to slide downwards into the bed, for that would be to produce one evil in curing another.

Sir Charles Bell thinks that the common disease of infants called *diabetes*, arises from their being permitted to sleep on their backs; and that by breaking up the habit of lying in this position, and accustoming them to lie on their sides, we shall prevent it. I doubt whether the effect here referred to, is ever the result of such a cause. Still I am as much opposed to the *habit* of sleeping on the back, as Sir Charles Bell. It is quite injurious to free respiration.

Closely allied to the subject of bodily position in general, is the state of particular organs; especially the stomach and the senses. I have already intimated that in order to have an infant sleep quietly, it is desirable to darken the room. This is the more necessary, where infants are unnaturally wakeful. In such cases, not only light should be excluded from the eye, but sounds from the ear, odors from the nostrils, &c. A remarkably full stomach is in the way of going quietly to sleep, whether the person be old or young. Neither infants nor adults ought to take food for some time previous to their going to sleep for the night. Great bodily heat, as well as too great cold, is also unfavorable. If too hot, the temperature of the infant should be somewhat reduced by exposure to the air; if too cold, it should be raised in a natural, healthy, and appropriate manner.

## SEC. 8. *State of the Mind.*

In giving directions how to procure pleasant dreams, Dr. Franklin mentions as a highly important requisition, the possession of a quiet conscience. A wise prescription, no doubt.

But infants, as well as adults, in order to sleep quietly, should have their minds and feelings in a state of tranquillity. The youngest child has its "troubles;" and it is highly important, if not indispensable, to *healthy* sleep, that the mother take all reasonable pains to remove them before sleep is induced.

We sometimes hear about children crying themselves to sleep, as if it were a matter of no consequence; and sometimes, as if it were, on the contrary, rather desirable. But is the sleep of an adult satisfying, who goes to bed in trouble, and only sleeps because nature is so exhausted that she cannot bear the protracted watchfulness any longer? Why then should we expect it, in the case of the infant?

I know an excellent father who is so far from believing this doctrine, that he silences the cries of his child by the word of command—and believes that in so doing, he promotes both his health and his happiness. He would no more let him cry himself to sleep than he would let him cough himself to sleep; though both crying and coughing, in their places, may be and undoubtedly are salutary.

Whatever may be the age and circumstances of an individual, he ought to retire for rest with a cheerful mind. All anxiety about the future, all regret about the past, all plans even, in regard to the business or amusement of the morrow, should be kept wholly out of the mind. We should yield ourselves up to the arms of sleep with the same quietude as if life were finished, and we had nothing more to do or think of.

## SEC. 9. *Quality of Sleep.*

The soundness, as well as other qualities, of sleep, differs greatly in different individuals; and even in the same night, with the same individual in different circumstances. The first four or five hours of sleep are usually more sound than the remainder. Hardly anything will interrupt the repose of some persons during the early part of the night, while they awake afterwards at the slightest noise or movement—the chirping of a cricket, or the playing of a kitten.

In profound sleep, we probably dream very little, if at all; but in other circumstances, we are constantly disturbed by dreaming, and sometimes start and wake in the greatest anxiety or horror.

Nightmare is generally accompanied by dreams of the most distressing kind. We imagine a wild beast, or a serpent in pursuit of us; or a rock is detached from some neighboring cliff, and is about to roll upon and crush us; and yet all our efforts to fly are unavailing. We seem chained to the spot; but while in the very jaws of destruction, perhaps we awake, trembling, and palpitating, and weary, as if something of a serious nature had really happened.

In the case of nightmare, it is more than probable that we fall asleep with our stomachs too heavily loaded with food, or with a smaller quantity of that which is highly indigestible. Or it may sometimes arise from an improper position of the body, such as disturbs the action of the stomach or lungs, or of both these organs. Lying on the back, when we first go to sleep, is very apt to produce nightmare.

But distressing dreams often follow an evening of anxious cares, especially if those cares preyed upon us for the last half hour; and also after late suppers, even if they are light—and late reading. Hence the injunctions of the last section. Hence, too, the importance of taking our last meal two or three hours before sleep, and of engaging, during these hours, in cheerful conversation, and in the social and private duties of religion. Family and private worship, in the evening, are enjoined no less by philosophy than they are by christianity; and every young mother will do well to understand this matter, and train her offspring accordingly.

"That sleep from which we are easily roused, is the healthiest," says Macnish. "Very profound slumber partakes of the nature of apoplexy." I should say, rather, that a medium between the two extremes is healthiest. Profound apoplectic sleep, I am sure, is injurious; but that from which we are too easily roused cannot, it seems to me, be less so. Thus, I have often gone to sleep with a resolution to wake at a certain hour, or at the striking of the clock; and have found myself able to wake at the proposed time, almost without one failure in twenty instances where I have made the trial. But my sleep was obviously unsound, and certainly unsatisfying. The desire to awake at a certain moment or period, seemed to buoy me above the usual state of healthy sleep, and render me liable to awake at the slightest disturbance. Were it not for sacrificing the ease of others, it would be far better, in such cases, to rely upon some person to wake us, instead of charging our own minds with it.

The quality of our sleep will be greatly affected by the quantity. But this thought, if extended, would anticipate the subject of our next section; so easily does one thing, especially in physical education, run into or involve another. I will therefore, for the present, only say that if we confine ourselves to a smaller number of hours than is really required, our sleep becomes too sound to be quite healthy, as if nature endeavored to make up in quality, for want of due quantity. On the contrary, if we attempt to sleep longer than is really necessary to restore us, the quality of our sleep is not what it ought to be; for we do not sleep soundly enough.

The silence and darkness of the night tend to induce sleep of a better quality than the noise and activity of day. It is unquestionably desirable that children should be able to sleep, at least occasionally, without absolute quiet. And yet such sleep cannot be sufficiently sound to answer the purposes of health, if frequently repeated.

Hence it is, perhaps—at least in part—that the maxim has obtained currency, that one hour of sleep before midnight is worth two afterward. The comparison has probably been made between the quiet and darksome hours of evening and those which followed daybreak, when light, and music, and bustle conspire, as they should, to make us wakeful. No person can sleep as soundly and as effectually, when light reaches his closed eyes, and sounds strike his ears, as in darkness and silence. He may sleep, indeed, under almost any circumstances, when fatigue and exhaustion demand it; but never so profoundly as when in absolute abstraction of light, and complete quiet.

## SEC. 10. *Quantity.*

On this point much might be said, without exhausting the subject. But I have already observed that infants, when first born, require to sleep nearly their whole time. As they advance in years, the necessity for sleep; however, diminishes, until they come to maturity, when it remains for many years nearly stationary. In advanced age, the necessity for sleep again increases, till we reach the extremest old age, or what is usually called second childhood, when we again sometimes sleep nearly the whole time.

I have already remarked that much might be said on this subject; but I do not think that the present occasion requires it. If the suggestions which are made in the chapter on "Early Rising" should receive the attention I flatter myself they merit, I do not believe children would often sleep too long. If, on the contrary, they are suffered to lie late in the morning, and then sit up late in the evening, all healthful habits and tendencies will he so deranged or broken up, that nature, in her indications, will by no means prove the unerring guide which she is wont to do in other circumstances.

A few thoughts here, on the quantity of sleep required by the young after they approach maturity, may not be misplaced.

Jeremy Taylor thought that for a healthy adult, three hours in twenty-four were enough for all the purposes of sleep. Baxter thought four hours about a reasonable time; Wesley, six; Lord Coke and Sir Wm. Jones, seven; and Sir John Sinclair, eight. These were the *theories* of men who were all eminent for their learning, and most of them for their piety. How far their *practice* corresponded with their theories, we are not, in every instance, told.

But to come to the practice of several persons who have been distinguished in the world. General Elliot, one of the most vigorous men of his age, though living for his whole life on nothing but vegetables and water, and who at sixty-four had scarcely begun to feel the infirmities of old age, slept but four hours in twenty-four. Frederick the Great of Prussia, and the illustrious British surgeon, John Hunter, slept but five hours a day. Napoleon Bonaparte, for a great part of his life, slept only four hours; and Lord Brougham is said to require no more. Others, in numerous instances, require but six hours. But there are others still, who consume eight.

The conclusion—in my own mind—is, that with a good constitution and active habits, men may habituate themselves to very different quantities of sleep. Still I think that six hours are little enough for most persons; and if a child, on arriving at maturity, is not inclined to sleep much longer than that, I should not regard him as wasting time. Most persons, it appears to me, require six hours of sound sleep in twenty-four;—I mean between the ages of twenty and seventy.

Macnish is the most liberal modern writer I am acquainted with, in his allowance of time for sleep. Speaking of the wants of adults he says—"No person who passes only eight hours in bed can be said to waste his time in sleep." Yet he obviously contradicts himself on the very same page; for he says expressly, that when a person is young, strong and healthy, an hour or two less may be sufficient. But an hour or two less than eight hours reduces the amount to seven or six hours. And taking the whole period of life, to which he probably refers—say from eighteen to forty—into consideration, there is a very considerable difference between six hours and eight hours a day. If six hours are "sufficient," it cannot be right to sleep eight hours.

Let us here make a few estimates. If six hours are sufficient for sleep between the ages of eighteen and forty, he who sleeps eight hours a day, actually loses 16,060 hours—equal to nearly two whole years of life, or about two years and three quarters of time in which we are usually awake. This, in the meridian of life, is not a small waste. Permit it to every person now in the United States, and the sum total of wasted time to a single generation, would be 25,649,098 years—equal to the average duration of the lives of 854,970 persons. The value of this time, as a commodity in the market, at a low estimate—only forty dollars a year—would be over A THOUSAND MILLIONS of DOLLARS! And its value, for the purposes of mental and moral improvement, cannot be estimated except in ETERNITY!

Every young mother must derive from these considerations a motive to discourage all unnecessary waste of time in sleep; while no one, as I trust, will forget that to sleep too little is also dangerous to health, and prejudicial to the general happiness.

# CHAPTER XV.

## EARLY RISING.

*All children naturally early risers. Evils of sitting up late at night. Excitements in the evening. The morning, by its beauties, invites us abroad. Example of parents. Forbidding children to rise early. Keeping them out of the way. How many are burnt up by parental neglect. "Lecturing" them. What is an early hour?*

Some writer—I do not recollect who—has said that all children are naturally early risers. And I cannot help coming to the same conclusion. That they are not so, is no more proved from the fact that as things now are they are generally found addicted to the contrary habit, than the very general neglect of milk among the higher classes of our citizens, proves that they have not a natural relish for it—when every one knows that at our first setting out in life, milk is, almost without exception, the sole article of human sustenance.

One of the great difficulties in the way of early rising, as I have already had occasion to say, is late sitting up. If children are not accustomed to retire till nine or ten o'clock, nor then until they have been subjected to all the excitements pertaining to fashionable life—company, heated and impure air, stimulating drink, fruits, high-seasoned food, and perhaps music—and are become actually feverish, no one but an ignorant person or a brute ought to expect them to rise early. Indeed, whatever may have been the cause, and whether it have operated on high or low life, late retiring will inevitably result in late rising. The current may be turned out of its course a little while, it is true, but not always. It will ere long return to its accustomed channel; perhaps to renew its course with increased pertinacity.

Everything, in the morning, naturally invites to early rising. The pleasant light, the music, at certain seasons, of some of the animated tribes, and the joy which we feel in activity, and in the society of those whom we love, all conspire to rouse us. If we have retired late, however, and especially in a feverish condition, so that when we wake we feel wretched, and, as sometimes happens, more fatigued than when we lay down, other collateral motives may be needed.

I have said that everything invites us, in the morning, to rise early; but it was upon the presumption that our parents, and brothers, and sisters set us a good example. If parents and other friends lie in bed late themselves, can anything else be, expected of children? Admitting, even, that they rise early themselves, if they never speak of early rising as a pleasure, and connect along with it, in their children's minds, pleasant associations, they would be unreasonable to expect otherwise than that their children should cling to the morning couch, till they are fairly compelled to rise as a relief from pain and uneasiness.

But when parents go farther than this, and actually discourage their children from rising early, and use every means in their power short of actual punishment—and sometimes even that—to make them lie still till breakfast, in order that they may be out of the way, what shall we say? And what is to be expected as the result?

There is hope, however, under the last circumstances. People sometimes carry things to an extreme that defeats their very purposes. Thus it occasionally is, in the case before us. This forbidding children to rise early, and threatening them if they do, sometimes excites their curiosity, and leads them to the forbidden course of conduct, simply *because* it is forbidden. Not a few persons among us possess the disposition to be governed by what has sometimes been called the "rule of contrary."

I might stop here to show that there is nothing so well calculated to develope and improve the mind and heart, even of parents themselves, as the society of those whom God gives them to train for Him and their country. I might show that not a few of those traits of character which render the company of many old persons rather irksome, especially to the young, have their origin in their neglect of the young, and of keeping up, as long as circumstances will possibly admit, juvenile feelings, actions, and habits.

And yet what do we too often witness in life? Is not every effort made to induce the young to lie in bed late that they may be out of the way? Are they not placed, as soon as possible after they are up, with the servants—if unfortunately there are any in the family—that they may be out of the way? Are they not required to breakfast, and dine, and sup elsewhere, if possible, that they may be out of the way? Do we not send them to school, even the Sabbath school, to get them out of the way? Do not some mothers even dose their infants with stupifying medicines to lull them to sleep, in order to have them out of the way? And to crown all, though they are quite too often permitted to sit up late in the evening, to enjoy that society which they are denied so great a part of the day-time, are they not occasionally put to bed early that they may be out of the way, and that the parents may attend late parties, to indulge in immoral or unhealthy habits?

In the last instance, they are indeed sometimes put out of the way, in the result—and with a vengeance. Many a child, nay, many thousands of children, are burnt up yearly, while their parents are gone abroad in the evening in quest of that enjoyment which ought to be found in the bosom of their families. "In Westminster, a part of London, containing less than two hundred thousand inhabitants, one hundred children were thus destroyed, during a single year." And the moral results which occasionally happen are a thousand times worse than burning. But enough of this.

The common practice of lecturing the young on the importance of early rising, may have a good effect on a few; but in general, it is believed to produce the contrary result. It is, in short, to sum up the whole matter, the influence of parental example, and the speaking often of the happiness which early rising affords, with perhaps the occasional indulgence of the child in a pleasant morning walk, which, if he retires early enough, are almost certain to produce in him the valuable habit of early rising.

But what is an early hour? Some call it early, when the sun is one hour high; some at sunrise; others, when they hear of an early riser, suppose he must be one who rises at least by daybreak.

Midnight is, of course, as near the middle of the night as any hour; and he who goes to bed four or five hours before midnight, will never complain of those who insist that *he* is not an early riser who is not up by four or five o'clock. In summer, no adult ought to lie in bed after four o'clock, and no child, except the mere infant, after five.

# CHAPTER XVI.

## HARDENING THE CONSTITUTION.

Mistakes about hardening children. Their clothing. Much cold enfeebles. The Scotch Highlanders. The two extremes equally fatal—over-tenderness and neglect. An interesting anecdote from Dr. Dewees.

While I have been very particular in enjoining on my readers the importance of thoroughly ventilating their dwellings, I have also insisted upon the necessity of taking children abroad, as much as possible. Not, however, to harden them, so much as to give them a more free access to air and light than they can have at home; and also—when they are old enough—to cultivate the faculties of attention, comparison, &c.

The practice of attempting to harden children by frequent exposure to air much colder than that to which they have been accustomed, without sufficient additional clothing, is open to the same objections which have been brought against cold bathing. Under the management of a judicious medical practitioner, it may do great good to a few constitutions; but its indiscriminate use would injure a thousand infants for one who was benefited.

True it is that if the child is protected against cold, no harm, but on the contrary much good may result, from carrying him abroad into the fresh air, even in very cold weather. But what can be more painful than to see the little sufferers carried along when their limbs are purple, or benumbed with cold? And how idle it is to hope that such exposure hardens or improves the constitution!

It is on the same mistaken principle that many adults go thinly clad, late in the fall. I have seen men in November and December beating and rubbing their hands, who, on being asked why they did not wear mittens, replied, that if they should wear one pair of mittens so early in the season, they should want two in the winter.

Now I cheerfully admit that to put on additional clothing before the severity of the weather demands it, actually produces the effect here supposed; but to endure severe cold, on the contrary, never hardens anybody. Nay, more, it enfeebles. Cold, when combined with the evils of *poverty*, produces more mischief and destroys more lives than any one disease in the whole catalogue of human maladies.

Adam Smith says that it is not uncommon for mothers in the Highlands of Scotland, who have borne twenty children, to have only two of them alive.

It may be difficult to say whether children are oftener destroyed by over-tenderness than by neglect, and the evils incident to poverty. Both extremes are common; while the happy medium—that of conducting a child's education upon the principles of physiology, is rarely known, and still more rarely followed.

I have been much amused, and not a little instructed, by the following anecdote on this point, from Dr. Dewees:

We were speaking with a lady who had lost three or four children with "croup," who informed us she was convinced, from absolute experiment, that there was nothing like exposure to all kinds of weather to protect and harden the system. By her first plan of managing her children, which was by keeping them very warmly clad, she said she lost several by the croup; but since she had adopted the opposite scheme, her children had been perfectly healthy, and never had betrayed the slightest disposition to that terrible disease which had robbed her of her children.

Perhaps, madam, we observed, you did not, in making your first experiments, attend to a number of details which might be thought essential to the plan. You did not probably take the proper precautions when you sent them into the cold air, or observe what was important for them when they returned from it.

"Oh, yes," she replied, "I took every possible care when they, were going out. I always made them wear a very warm great coat, well lined with baize, and a fur cape or collar. I always made them wear a 'comfortable' round their necks, made of soft woollen yarn. And as for their feet, they were always protected by socks or over-shoes lined with wool or fur, as the weather might be wet or dry."

Do you believe, madam, they were kept at a proper degree of warmth by these means?

"Oh, certainly. Indeed, rather too warm; for they would often be in a state of perspiration, they told me, when in the open air; especially if they ran, slid, or skated."

And what was done when they were thus heated?

"Oh, they got cool enough before they reached home."

And would they receive no injury in passing from this state of perspiration to that of chill?

"Not at all; for when this happened, I always made them take a little warm brandy, or wine and water, and made them toast their feet well by the fire." [Footnote: This absurd custom is a fruitful source of that distressing condition of the hands and feet, in winter, called "chilblains."]

Did they sleep in a cold or warm room?

"In a warm room. A good fire was always made in the stove before they went to bed, which kept them quite warm all night."

Would they never complain of being cold towards morning, when the stove had become cold?

"Yes, certainly; but then there were always at hand additional bed-clothes, with which they could cover themselves."

And did they always do it?

"Oh, I suppose so."

Well, madam, how did you carry your second plan into execution, which you say was attended with such happy results?

"I began by not letting them put on their great coats, except when the weather was so cold as to require this additional covering, and did not permit them to wear a 'comfortable' or fur round their necks. I took away their over-shoes, and if their feet chanced to get wet, (for they were always provided with good sound shoes,) the shoes were immediately changed, if they were at home. If the weather was wet, or unusually cold, they were permitted to wear their great coats, but not without. If they came home very cold, they were not allowed to approach the fire too soon. I gave them no warm, heating drinks, and accustomed them to sleep in rooms without fire."

Who does not recognize, in this second plan for the enjoyment of air and exercise, as judicious a plan of physical education, so far as it goes, as can well be pointed out? We were so successful as to convince this lady, in a very short time, that our own plan of exposing the body was precisely the one she had pursued with so much success.

We also inquired of her what plan she pursued with her children, when too young to be submitted to the rules just mentioned. She informed us that it was the same system throughout, only the details varied as circumstances of age, &c. made it necessary. That is, she sent her children into the open air at very early periods of their lives, provided in summer it was neither too wet nor too warm; in winter, when the air was mild, dry and clear—but always carefully wrapped up, that their little extremities might not suffer from cold. She never suffered them to sleep in the open air, if it could be avoided; to prevent which, as much as possible, she constantly charged the nurse to bring the children home, as soon as she found them disposed to sleep, unless it was when they were very young, at which time it was impossible to guard against it.

And when her children were sufficiently old to walk, she took care to prepare them properly for it, whether it might be in warm, cold, or moderate weather. She never sent them abroad for pleasure at the risk of encountering a storm of any kind; nor permitted them to walk at the hazard of getting wet or very muddy feet.

Were the constitutions of your children pretty much the same? we demanded of this lady.

"No; one of my boys was extremely feeble, from his very birth."

# CHAPTER XVII.

## SOCIETY.

*Duty of mothers in this matter. Children prefer the society of parents. Importance of other society. Necessity of society illustrated. Early diffidence. Selecting companions for children. Moral effects of society on the young. Parents should play with their children.*

Every mother is unquestionably as much bound to have an eye to the society of her child, as to his food, drink or clothing. And if the quality, amount and general character of the latter are important, those of the former are by no means less so.

It is indeed true that many a child has been happy, in a degree, in the society of its mother alone, where the father was seldom seen, and the brothers and sisters never. And it is equally true; that a few children have so far preferred the society of their parents alone, as to become disinclined to other society. But cases of this kind are only as exceptions to the general rule; and are probably monstrous formations of character. I cannot believe that any child, rightly educated, would prefer the society of none but its parents, or even its parents and brothers and sisters.

A French author has written a considerable volume on the importance of what he calls *gaiety*, but which he should prefer to call cheerfulness. Among the rest, he maintains that it is indispensable to the best health. But if so—and I do not doubt it—then it ought to be encouraged in children, and the earlier the better. Now there is no way to encourage cheerfulness in the young so effectually as by indulging them with considerable society.

That the thing may be carried to excess, I have no doubt. I have seen mothers who permitted their children to play with their mates till they became excited, and were thus led to continue their sports, not only farther than cheerfulness and health demanded, but until they were excessively fatigued, and almost made sick. And I believe that the excitement of numbers, in infant and other schools, may be so great as to be injurious, rather than salutary. Still I think these are rare cases.

Truth usually lies somewhere between extremes. To keep a child, especially a boy, always in the nursery, or even in the parlor with his mother, is one extreme; and to let him go abroad continually, till his home and its smaller circle become insipid, is the other. A child properly trained will *usually* prefer home, and only desire to go abroad occasionally. He will rather need urging in the matter than require restraint.

But he must, at any rate, be taught to be sociable, not only for the salve of cheerfulness and the consequent health, but for the sake of his manners, his mind, and his morals.

If it is a matter of indifference, in the formation of human character, whether we mix in society or not, then, for anything I can see, an improvement might be proposed in the construction of the material universe. Instead of forming the planets so large—and this earth among the rest—each might have been divided into hundreds of millions; and every human being might have had a little planet, and an immortality, exclusively his own. Such an arrangement would certainly prevent a great many evils; and, among the rest, a great deal of quarrelling and bloodshed.

But divine wisdom is higher than human wisdom, and one world to hundreds of millions of human beings has been made, instead of giving to each individual of the universe a little world of his own, in which he might have reigned sole monarch, and only wept, with Alexander, because none of the other worlds were within his grasp. Where a family is already large, other society will be unnecessary for some time; but where it consists of a mother only, although her society is always to be considered of the *first* importance, I cannot but think she ought to take great pains to introduce her child occasionally to the company of other children.

That diffidence, which almost destroys the influence and the happiness of many individuals, is often cherished, if not created, by too much seclusion. Where there is a natural constitution which predisposes the child to timidity and diffidence, the danger is greatly increased; and parents should take unwearied pains to guard against it.

It is hardly necessary for me to say, that great care should also be used in selecting the companions of children. Their character will be greatly influenced for life by their earlier associates. Friendships between children are sometimes formed, while playing together, which are interrupted only by death. Those parents who are so fond of controlling the choice of their sons and daughters in regard to a companion for life, at a period when control is generally resisted, would do well to take a hint from what has here been suggested. There is no doubt but they might often—very often—give such a direction to the embryo affections of their infants and children, as would terminate only with their existence.

It is still less necessary to advert, in a work like this, to the effect which much observation and experience shows good society to have on purity, both physical and moral. Every one must have observed its tendency to form habits of cleanliness, not to say neatness. There may be excess, even in this. Young persons, of both sexes, often spend too much time in preparing their dress for the reception or the visiting of their friends. Still this is only the abuse of a good thing. Nor is it less true, though it may be less obvious, that moral purity is more likely to be secured where children and youth of both sexes associate a great deal, from the earliest infancy. [Footnote: If this principle be correct, what is the tendency of our numerous schools, which are exclusively for one sex? Must there not be latent evil to counterbalance some of the seeming good? For myself, I doubt whether moral character can ever be formed in due proportion and harmony, where this separation long exists.] There are tremendous cases of declension on record, which establish this point beyond the possibility of debate.

To say that the mother—and indeed both parents—ought to form a part of the playing circle of the youngest children, in order to watch their opening dispositions, to check what may be improper, and encourage what ought to be encouraged, would be only to repeat what has often been recommended by the best writers on education—but which must be repeated, again and again, till it leaves an impression, especially on CHRISTIAN parents. It is strange that many regard this matter as they do, and appear not only ashamed to be seen sporting with their children, but almost ashamed to have their children thus occupied. They might as well be ashamed of the gambols of the kitten or the lamb; or of the grave mother, as she turns aside occasionally to join in its frolics.

# CHAPTER XVIII.

## EMPLOYMENTS.

Influence of mothers over daughters. Anecdote of Benjamin West. Anecdote of a poor mother. Of set lessons and lectures. Daughters under the mother's eye. Why young ladies, now-a-days, dislike domestic employments. Miserable housewives —not to be wondered at. Mistake of one class of men. Mr. Flint's opinion.

One important and never-to-be-forgotten employment of the young is the cultivation of their minds; and another, that of their morals. But my present purpose is only to speak of those employments denominated manual, or physical.

It is obvious, at the first glance, that the influence of the mother, in our own country, at least, will be less over boys than over girls. We leave it to savages and semi-savages to employ their females, and even their mothers, in hard manual labor. Here, in America, what I should say on the employment of boys would be more properly addressed to the YOUNG FATHER.

There are some exceptions to the general truth contained in the last paragraph. Many a mother has—unconsciously at the time, but with no less certainty than if she had done it intentionally—given a direction to the whole current of her son's life; and this, too, at a very early period. The mother of Benjamin West, the painter, if she did not give the first tendency to his favorite pursuit, while he was yet a mere child, at the least greatly confirmed him in it, by the manner of expressing her surprise at one of his early performances. "My mother's kiss," on that occasion, said he, "made me a painter." Nor are facts of the same general character by any means uncommon.

I know a poor mother who, in the absence of her husband at his weekly or monthly labors, used to detain her eldest boy, then almost an infant, from going to bed in the evening till her day's work was finished—because, in her loneliness, she wanted his company—by telling stories of eminent men, and especially of distinguished philanthropists, until she had unconsciously kindled in him a philanthropic spirit, which will not cease to burn till his death.

But it is in forming the predilections of daughters for their destined employments, that mothers are especially influential. Not so much by their set lessons or lectures, however, as by the force of continued example. No mother who sends her child away to be nursed, and subsequently to her return seizes on every possible opportunity to keep her out of the way and out of her sight, will be likely to give her any choice of employment, or indeed any fondness for employment at all.

Nor is it sufficient that she keep her daughter constantly under her eye, with a view to qualify her for the duties of a housewife, if the daughter see as plainly as in the light of mid-day, that the mother dislikes the employment herself. She must love what she would have her daughter love, and even what she would have her understand. Nor is it sufficient that she *affect* a fondness for the employment; her love for it must be real. Little girls have keener eyes and better judgments than some mothers seem willing to believe or to admit.

Many persons seem greatly surprised that the young ladies of modern days have so little fondness for domestic life and domestic duties. How few, it is often said, will do their own housework, if they can possibly get a train of domestics around them; even though the care and oversight of the domestics themselves gear them out more rapidly than bodily labor would.

But there is a reason for this hostility to domestic employments. It is because mothers, almost universally, consider their occupations as mere drudgery, and bring up their children in the same spirit. And what else could be expected as the result? It would be an anomaly in the history, of human nature, if the female members of families were to grow up in love with ordinary domestic avocations, when they have been accustomed to see their mothers, and nurses, and elder sisters complaining and fretting while engaged in them; and showing by their actions, no less than by their words, that they regarded themselves as miserable and wretched.

No wonder so many girls, of the present day, make miserable housewives. No wonder a factory, a book-bindery, or a shoemaker's shop, is considered preferable to the kitchen. No wonder the world degenerates, because females, no longer healthfully employed, become pale and sickly, spreading gloom and misery all around them, and transmitting the same ills which themselves suffer to those who come after them.

It is true, the guilt of this dereliction must not be charged wholly on mothers; though they ought, unquestionably, to bear a large share of it. Those who have, and ought to have, much influence in society, erroneously, and I suppose thoughtlessly, help mothers along in their evil ways. If there were a universal combination between certain classes of mankind and the whole race of mothers, to ruin, rather than be instrumental of reforming mankind, and of saving their deathless souls, I hardly know how they could invent a much better, or at least a much more certain plan, than that now in operation. So long as those who take the lead in society, and govern the fashion in this matter, as others govern it in the matter of dress, refuse, as a general rule, to form alliances for life, except with those who practically despise house-hold concerns—and so long as our houses are filled with domestics, whose object is to aid these spoiled mothers, but whose real effect is to complete their ruin, and accelerate the ruin of mankind—just so long will human progress towards perfection be retarded.

If mothers were in love with their occupations, and their daughters knew it, then to the influence of a good example they could add many lessons of instruction. These might be given in the way of natural, unstudied conversation, and thus be not only heard with attention, but sink deep. If the world is ever to be reformed, says Mr. Flint, in his Western Review, woman, sensible, enlightened, well educated and principled, must be the original mover in the great work. Every one who has considered well the extent and nature of female influence, will concur in the sentiment; and if he have one remaining particle of devotion to the Father of spirits, he will send up the most fervent petitions to his throne of mercy in behalf of this often depressed or enslaved half of the human race, that they may speedily be emancipated, and become as conspicuous in human redemption, as they have sometimes been in human condemnation.

# CHAPTER XIX.

## EDUCATION OF THE SENSES.

Improving the senses. Examples of improvement. SEC. 1. Hearing—how injured—how improved.—SEC. 2. Seeing—how injured.—SEC. 3. Tasting and smelling—how benumbed—how preserved.—SEC. 4. Feeling. The blind. Hints to parents. Education of both hands.

Man is much less useful and happy in this world than he would be, if more pains were taken by parents and teachers, as well as by himself, to cultivate his senses—hearing, seeing, feeling; tasting, and smelling—and to preserve their rectitude.

The extent to which the senses can be improved or exalted, can best be understood by observing how perfect they become when we are compelled to cultivate them. Thus the blind, who are obliged to cultivate hearing, feeling, and smelling, often astonish us by the keenness of these senses. They will distinguish sounds—especially voices—which others cannot; and with so much accuracy, as to remember for several years the voice of a person in a large company, which they hear but once. They will also distinguish small pieces of money, different fabrics and qualities of cloth, &c.; and, in walking, often ascertain, by the feeling of the air, or by other sensations, when they approach a building, or any other considerable body. So the North American Indian, whose habits of life seem to require it, can hear the footsteps of an approaching enemy at distances which astonish us. So also the deaf and dumb are very keen-sighted, and generally make very accurate observations. Any reader who is sceptical in regard to the cultivation of the senses, would do well to consult the account of Julia Brace, the deaf and dumb and blind girl, as published in some of the early volumes of the "Annals of Education."

But it is hardly necessary to resort to the blind, or to savages, or to the deaf and dumb, in order to prove man's susceptibility in this respect. We may be reminded of the same fact by observing with what accuracy the merchant tailor can distinguish, by feeling, the quality of his goods; how quick a painter, an engraver, or a printer, will discover errors in painting or printing, which wholly escape ordinary readers or observers; and how quick the ear of a good musician will discover the existence and origin of a discordant sound in his choir.

Now I do not undertake to say or prove, that mankind would be better or happier for having their senses all cultivated in the highest possible degree; though I am not sure that this would not be the case. But so long as a large proportion of our ideas enter our minds through the medium of the five senses, it is desirable that something should be done to perfect them, instead of overlooking the whole subject. What mothers ought to do in this matter, deserves, therefore, a brief consideration.

## SEC. 1. *Hearing.*

The suggestion, in another place, to keep away caps from the child's head, if duly attended to, is one means of perfecting, or at least of preserving, the sense of hearing. For caps, by the heat they produce to a part which cannot safely endure an increase of temperature, greatly expose children to catarrhal affections; and many a catarrh has laid the foundation for dulness of hearing, if not of actual deafness.

The ears should be kept clean. If washed sufficiently often, and syringed once a week with warm milk and water, or with very weak soap-suds, gently warmed, the cerumen or ear wax will hardly be found accumulated in such masses as to produce deafness. And yet such accumulations, with such consequences, are by no means uncommon. It is not long since a young man with whom I am acquainted, applied to an eminent surgeon of Boston, on account of deafness in one ear, which had become quite troublesome, and as it was feared, incurable. Syringing with a large and strong syringe disengaged a large mass of cerumen, and hearing was immediately restored.

Children should be taught to distinguish sounds with closed eyes, or blindfolded. We may strike on various objects, and ask them to tell what we struck, &c. This will lead them to *observe* sounds; and will perfect their hearing in a remarkable degree.

There are also advantages to be derived from accustoming a child to a great variety of sounds; both as regards their strength and character. But this must only be occasional; for if the ear be constantly accustomed to sounds of any kind, and more especially those which are harsh or loud, the organ of hearing is liable to sustain injury. Music, as it is now beginning to be taught to children in our schools, will do much, I think, to improve the faculty of hearing.

### SEC. 2. *Seeing.*

The sight, says Addison, is the most perfect of all our senses; and this is unquestionably true. But it is more or less perfect, in different individuals, according to the early education they have received. Sometimes, it is true, we are born near-or dim-sighted; but such cases are comparatively rare.

The question is sometimes asked why there are so many persons, now-a-days, who lose their sight, become near-sighted, &c. very young. It may be difficult to answer this question fully; yet I cannot help thinking that the following are some of the causes.

1. The great heat of our apartments, which, together with late hours and much lamp light, affects the eyes unpleasantly, is believed to be among the more prominent causes of early decay of sight. Formerly, our apartments were neither so steadily nor so generally heated; and we rose earlier, and consequently went to bed earlier.

2. The fine print of a large proportion of our books, especially our school books, has done immense injury. I do not believe that reading fine print, occasionally, for a few moments at a time, or reading by a very strong or very weak light in the same way, does harm. On the contrary, I think it may strengthen and improve the sight. It is the long continuance of these things that does the mischief; and the mischief thus done is immense. I rejoice that

printers and publishers are beginning of late to use much larger type than they have done for some years past.

3. The early use of spectacles does mischief—I mean before they are needed. After they begin to be needed, there is no advantage in delaying to use them, as some do, for fear they shall wear them too soon. This is about as wise as the practice of going cold to harden ourselves.

4. Reading when we are fatigued, or ill, or have a very full stomach, is another way to injure the sight.

5. Rubbing the eyes with the fingers, or with anything else, does inevitable mischief. The Germans have a proverb which says—"Never touch your eye, except with your elbow." There is much of good sense in it.

In short, there are a thousand ways in which that delicate organ, the human eye, may sustain injury; and nearly as many in which it may be strengthened, cultivated, and improved. But my limits merely permit me to add, that the frequent but gentle application of water to the eye, several times a day, at such a temperature as is most agreeable—but cold, when it can be borne—is one of the best preservatives of sight which the world affords.

Connected alike with physical and intellectual education, is the practice of measuring by the eye heights, distances, superfices, weights, and solids. It is not difficult to train the eye to an accuracy in this matter which would astonish the uninstructed.

## SEC. 3. *Tasting and Smelling.*

I do not know that it is worth our while to take pains, by any direct methods, to cultivate the organs of taste or smell; but I think it proper, at the least, to preserve their original rectitude.

Many, I know, undertake to say, that were it not for our errors in regard to food and drink, and were it not, in particular, for the multitude of strange mixtures which tend to benumb those two senses, we might determine the qualities of food and drink—whether they are favorable or adverse—by means of taste and smell, like the animals. But I do not believe this. The Creator has substituted reason, in us, for instinct in the brute animals. It is not necessary that we should possess the latter, when the former is so manifestly superior to it; and accordingly I do not believe that it is given us, or any of that acuteness of sensation which exists in the dog, the tiger, the vulture, &c.—and which so closely resembles it.

There can be no doubt—no reasonable doubt, certainly—that the wretched customs of modern cookery benumb the senses of taste and smell, more or less, and that high-seasoned food, condiments, and stimulating drinks do the same; and should for this reason, were it for no other, be studiously avoided.

Closely connected with the organ of taste are the TEETH. A volume might profitably be written on these—as on the eye. But I will only say that they should be kept perfectly clean, either by rinsing or brushing, or both, especially after eating; that they should be permitted to chew all our food, instead of merely standing by as silent spectators to the passage of that which is mashed, soaked, chopped, &c.; that they should not be picked or cleaned with pins, or other equally hard instruments; that they should not be used to crack nuts or other hard, indigestible substances; and that the stomach, with which they are apt to sympathize very strongly, should also be kept in a good and healthy condition.

### SEC. 4. *Feeling.*

Corpulence and slovenliness are generally among the more prolific sources of a want of acuteness in feeling. The first is a disease, and may be avoided by a proper diet, and by active mental and bodily employment. Slovenliness we may of course avoid, whenever there is a wish to do so, and an abundance of water.

But the sense of feeling, or especially that accumulation of it which we call TOUCH, and which seems to be specially located in the balls of the fingers and on the palm of the hand, is susceptible of a degree of improvement far beyond what would be the natural result of cleanliness, and freedom from plethora or corpulence.

I have already alluded, in my general remarks at the head of this chapter, to the acuteness of this sense in the blind, as well as in the dealer in cloths. I might add many more illustrations, but a single one, in relation to the blind, which was accidentally omitted in that place, will be sufficient.

The blind at the Institution in this city, as well as in other similar institutions, are now taught to read and write with considerable facility. But how? Most of my readers may have heard how they read, but I will describe the process as well as I can. A description of their method of writing is more difficult.

The letters are formed by pressing the paper, while quite moist, upon rather large type, which raises a ridge in the line of every letter, and which remains prominent after the paper is dry. In order to read, the pupil has to feel out these ridges. A circular ridge on the paper he is told is O; a perpendicular one, I; a crooked one, S; &c. They read music and arithmetic printed in a similar manner. A few months of practice, in this way, will enable an ingenious youth to read with considerable ease and despatch.

Now if nothing is wanting but a little training to render the touch so accurate, would it not be useful to train every child to judge frequently of the properties of bodies by this sense? And cannot every one recall to his mind a thousand situations in which a greater accuracy of this sense would have saved him much inconvenience, as well as afforded him no little pleasure?

I shall conclude this section with a few remarks on the HAND. The custom of neglecting, or almost neglecting the left hand, though nearly universal, in this country at least, appears to me to be wrong—decidedly so. For although more blood may be sent to the right arm than to the left, as physiologists say, yet the difference is not as great at birth as it is afterward; so that education either weakens the one or strengthens the other.

Besides this, we occasionally find a person who is left-handed, as it is called; that is, his left hand and arm are as much larger and stronger than the right, as the right is usually stronger than the left. How is this? Do we find a corresponding change in the internal structure? But suppose it could be ascertained that such a change did exist, which I believe has never been done, the question would still arise whether the difference was the same at birth, or whether the more frequent use of the left hand has not, in part, produced it.

I do not mean, here, to intimate that a more frequent use of the left hand than the right would make new blood-vessels grow where there were none before. But it would certainly do one thing; it would make the same vessels carry more blood than they did before, which is, in effect, nearly the same thing:—for the more blood in the limb, as a general rule, the more strength —provided the limb is in due health and exercise.

The inference which I wish the reader to make from all this is, that since the left hand and arm, by due cultivation, and without essential difference or change of structure to begin with, can occasionally be made stronger than the right, it is fair to conclude that it may, if found desirable, be always rendered more nearly equal to it than, in adult years, we usually find it.

The question is now fairly before us—Is such a result desirable? I maintain that it is; and shall endeavor to show my reasons.

How often is one hand injured by an accident, or rendered nearly useless by disease? But if it should be the right, how helpless it makes us! The man who is accustomed to shave himself, must now resort to a barber. If he is a barber himself, or almost any other mechanic, his business must be discontinued. Or if he is a clerk, he cannot use his left hand, and must consequently lose his time. Or if amputation chances to be performed on a favorite arm, how entirely useless to society we are, till we have learned to use the other! It not only takes up a great deal of valuable time to acquire a facility of using it, but if we are already arrived at maturity, we can never use it so well as the other, during our whole lives; because it is too late in life to increase its size and strength much by constant exercise. Whereas in youth, it might have been done easily.

# CHAPTER XX.

## ABUSES.

Bad seats for children at table and elsewhere. Why children hate Sunday. Seats at Sabbath school—at church—at district schools. Suspending children between the heavens and the earth. Cushions to sit on. Seats with backs. Children in factories. Evils produced. Bodily punishment. Striking the heads of children very injurious. Beating across the middle of the body. Anecdote of a teacher. Concluding advice to mothers.

It is difficult to determine, in regard to many things which concern the management of the young, whether they belong most properly to moral or physical education; so close is the connection between the two, and so decidedly does everything, or nearly everything which relates to the management of the body, have a bearing upon the formation of moral character. This work might be extended very much farther, did it comport with my original plan. But I hasten to close the volume, with a few thoughts on certain abuses of the body, which prevail to a greater or less extent in families and schools; and to which I have not adverted elsewhere.

The seats of children are usually bad, both at table and elsewhere. It seems not enough that we condemn them to the use of knives, forks, spoons, &c., of the same size with those of adults. We go farther; and give them chairs of the same height and proportion with our own. There are a few exceptions to the truth of this remark. Here and there we see a child's chair, it is true—but not often.

But how unreasonable is it to seat a child in a chair so high that his feet cannot reach the floor; and so constructed that there is no outer place on which the feet can rest. What adult would be willing to sit in so painful a posture, with his legs dangling? No wonder children dislike to sit much, in such circumstances. And it is a great blessing to both parent and child that they do. No wonder children hate the Sabbath, especially in those families where they are compelled to keep the day holy by sitting motionless!

Sabbath schools, though they bring with them some evil along with a great deal of good, are a relief to the young in this particular—especially if their seats are more comfortable elsewhere than at home. They consider it much more tolerable to spend the morning and intermission of the day in going and returning from Sabbath school, than in constant and close confinement. They prefer variety, and the occasional light and air of heaven, to monotony and seclusion and silence.

It happens, however, that the seats at the Sabbath school and at church, are not always what they should be; nor, so far as church is concerned, do I see that this evil can be wholly avoided. Children usually sit with their parents, in the sanctuary—and they ought to do so: and the height of the seats cannot, of course, accommodate both. If there is a building erected solely for the use of the Sabbath school, the seats may be constructed accordingly, without seriously incommoding anybody; but in the church, I do not see, as I have once before observed, how the evil can be remedied.

The greatest trouble in regard to seats, however, is at the day school; especially in our district or common schools. There, it is usual for children to be confined six hours a day—and sometimes two in succession—to hard, narrow, plank seats, a large proportion of which are without backs, and raised so high that the feet of most of the pupils cannot possibly touch the floor. There, "suspended," as I have said in another work, [Footnote: See a "Prize Essay," on School Houses, page 7.] "between the heavens and the earth, they are compelled to remain motionless for an hour or an hour and a half together."

I have also shown, in the same essay, that in regard to the desks, and indeed many other things which pertain to, or are connected with the school, very little pains is taken to provide for the physical welfare or even comfort of the pupils; and that a thorough reform on the subject appears to be indispensable.

When I speak of hard plank seats, let me not be understood as hinting at the necessity of cushions. When I wrote the essay above mentioned, I did indeed believe that they were desirable. But I am now opposed to their use, either by children or adults, even where a laborious employment would seem to demand a long confinement to this awkward and unnatural position. If our seats are cushioned, we shall sit too easily. I believe that our health requires a hard seat; because its very hardness inclines us to change, frequently, our position.

But if we must sit, be it ever so short a time, our seats should always have backs; and those which are designed for children, should not be so high as to render them uncomfortable. Nor should the backs of seats be so high as they usually are, either for children or adults. They should never come much higher than the middle of the body. If they reach the shoulders, they either favor a crouching forward, or interfere with the free action of the lungs.

This might be deemed a proper place for saying something on the position of children in manufactories. But here a world of abuse opens upon my view, the full development of which demands a large volume. How many crooked spines, emaciated bodies, decaying lungs, as well as scrofulas, fevers, and consumptions, are either induced or accelerated by these unnatural employments! I mean they are unnatural for the *young*. As to employing adults in them, I have nothing at present to say. But when I think of the cruel custom of placing children in these places, whose bodies —and were this the place, I might add, *minds*—are immature, and especially girls, I am compelled, by the voice of conscience, and, as I trust, by a regard to those laws which God has established in our physical frames, but which are yet so strangely violated, to protest against it. Better that no factories should exist, than that children should be ruined in them as they now are. Better by far that we should return, were it possible, to the primitive habits of New England—to those by-gone days when mothers and daughters made the wearing apparel of themselves and their families— when, if there was less of intellectual cultivation, and less money expended for luxuries and extravagances, there was much more of health and happiness.

There is one more species of abuse to which, in closing, I wish to direct maternal attention. I allude to injudicious modes of inflicting corporal punishment.

Let me not be understood to appear, in this place, as the advocate of bodily punishments of any kind; for if they are even admissible under some circumstances, I am fully convinced that in the way in which they are commonly administered, they do much more harm than good.

But leaving the question of their utility, in the abstract, wholly untouched, and taking it for granted, for the present, that they are—as is undoubtedly the fact—sometimes employed, and will continue to be so for a great while to come, I proceed to speak of their more flagrant abuses.

Among these, none are more reprehensible than blows of any kind on the head. Even the rod is objectionable for this purpose, since it exposes the eyes. But the hand—in boxing the ears or striking in any way—is more so. The bones of the head, in young children, are not yet firmly knit together, and these concussions may injure the tender brain. I know of whole families, whose mental faculties are dull, as the consequence—I believe—of a perpetual boxing and striking of the head. Some individuals are made almost idiots, in this very manner.—But the worst is not yet told. Many teachers are in the habit of striking their pupils' heads with thick heavy books; and with wooden rules. I have seen one of the latter, of considerable size and thickness, broken in two across the head of a very small boy; and this, too—such is the public mind—in the presence of a mother who was paying a visit to the school. I have seen parents and masters strike the heads of their children with pieces of wood, of much larger size;—in one instance with a common sized tailor's press-board; in another with the heavy end of a wooden whip-handle, about an inch in diameter.

Children are sometimes severely beaten across the middle of the body—the region where lie the vital organs—the lungs, the heart, the liver, &c. They are sometimes beaten too, across the joints, or in any place that the excited, perhaps passionate teacher or parent can reach. Rules and books are thrown with violence at pupils in school. There is a story in the "Annals of Education," Vol. IV. at page 28, of a teacher who threw a rule at a little boy, six years old, which struck him with great force, within an inch of one of his eyes. Had it struck a little nearer to his nose, it would, in all probability, have destroyed his left eye.

But without extending these remarks any farther, every intelligent mother who reads what I have already written, will see, as I trust, the necessity of properly informing herself on the great subject of physical education; and of being better prepared than she has hitherto been for acquitting herself, with satisfaction, of those high and sacred responsibilities which, in the wise arrangements of Nature and Providence, devolve upon her.